Positive Living with HIV/AIDS

Editors

KENNETH D. PHILLIPS
TERESA M. STEPHENS

NURSING CLINICS
OF NORTH AMERICA

www.nursing.theclinics.com

Consulting Editor
STEPHEN D. KRAU

March 2018 • Volume 53 • Number 1

ELSEVIER

1600 John F. Kennedy Boulevard • Suite 1800 • Philadelphia, Pennsylvania, 19103-2899

http://www.theclinics.com

NURSING CLINICS OF NORTH AMERICA Volume 53, Number 1
March 2018 ISSN 0029-6465, ISBN-13: 978-0-323-58162-2

Editor: Kerry Holland
Developmental Editor: Casey Potter

Nursing Clinics of North America (ISSN 0029-6465) is published quarterly by Elsevier Inc., 360 Park Avenue South, New York, NY 10010-1710. Months of issue are March, June, September, and December. Periodicals postage paid at New York, NY and additional mailing offices. Subscription price per year is, $155.00 (US individuals), $465.00 (US institutions), $275.00 (international individuals), $567.00 (international institutions), $220.00 (Canadian individuals), $567.00 (Canadian institutions), $100.00 (US students), and $135.00 (international students). To receive student/resident rate, orders must be accompanied by name of affiliated institution, date of term, and the signature of program/residency coordinator on institution letterhead. Orders will be billed at individual rate until proof of status is received. Foreign air speed delivery is included in all *Clinics* subscription prices. All prices are subject to change without notice. **POSTMASTER:** Send address changes to *Nursing Clinics*, Elsevier Health Sciences Division, Subscription Customer Service, 3251 Riverport Lane, Maryland Heights, MO 63043. **Customer Service: Telephone: 1-800-654-2452** (U.S. and Canada); **1-314-447-8871 (outside U.S. and Canada). Fax: 1-314-447-8029. E-mail: journalscustomerservice-usa@elsevier.com** (for print support) and **journalsonlinesupport-usa@elsevier.com** (for online support).

Nursing Clinics of North America is covered in *EMBASE/Excerpta Medica*, *MEDLINE/PubMed (Index Medicus)*, *Social Sciences Citation Index*, *Current Contents*, *ASCA*, *Cumulative Index to Nursing*, *RNdex Top 100*, and Allied Health Literature and International Nursing Index (INI).

Contributors

CONSULTING EDITOR

STEPHEN D. KRAU, PhD, RN, CNE
Associate Professor, Vanderbilt University Medical Center, School of Nursing, Nashville, Tennessee

EDITORS

KENNETH D. PHILLIPS, PhD, RN
Associate Dean for Research and Director of the PhD Program, College of Nursing, East Tennessee State University, Johnson City, Tennessee

TERESA M. STEPHENS, PhD, MSN, RN, CNE
Associate Professor, College of Nursing, Medical University of South Carolina, Charleston, South Carolina

AUTHORS

PRIYANKA AMIN, MD
Resident, Department of Psychiatry, Western Psychiatric Institute and Clinic of UPMC, Pittsburgh, Pennsylvania

MELINDA ANN BOGARDUS, RN, MSN, FNP-BC
Clinical Instructor, Walden University, College of Health Sciences, School of Nursing, Minneapolis, Minnesota; Doctoral Student, East Tennessee State University, College of Nursing, Johnson City, Tennessee; Family Nurse Practitioner, AppHealthCare, Jefferson, North Carolina

WILLIAM ANDREW CLARK, PhD, RD
Associate Dean of Research/Professor of Clinical Nutrition, The College of Clinical & Rehabilitative Health Sciences, East Tennessee State University, Johnson City, Tennessee

DAVID B. CLUCK, PharmD
Associate Professor, Department of Pharmacy Practice, East Tennessee State University, Bill Gatton College of Pharmacy, Johnson City, Tennessee

EILEEN M. CRESS, EdD, RD
Education/PI Dietitian, James H. Quillen VA Medical Center, Mountain Home, Tennessee

SABRA S. CUSTER, DNP, MS, FNP-BC
Clinical Associate Professor, College of Nursing, University of South Carolina, Columbia, South Carolina

AARON J. DIEHR, PhD, CHES
Chair, HIV/AIDS Section, American Public Health Association, Public Health and Recreation Professions, Southern Illinois University, Carbondale, Illinois

ANTOINE DOUAIHY, MD
Professor of Psychiatry and Medicine, University of Pittsburgh School of Medicine, Pittsburgh, Pennsylvania

KARL GOODKIN, MD, PhD, DFAPA, FACPsych
Professor and Chair, Department of Psychiatry and Behavioral Sciences, Quillen College of Medicine, East Tennessee State University, Johnson City, Tennessee

ROBIN HARRIS, PhD, ANP-BC, ACNS-BC
Clinical Assistant Professor, College of Nursing, The University of Tennessee, Knoxville, Knoxville, Tennessee

KYLEANNE HUNTER, PhD
Research Fellow, Josef Korbel School of International Studies, University of Denver, Denver, Colorado

JASON R. JAGGERS, PhD
Department of Health and Sport Sciences, University of Louisville, Louisville, Kentucky

STEVEN F. KENDELL, MD
Associate Professor, Department of Psychiatry and Behavioral Sciences, Quillen College of Medicine, East Tennessee State University, Johnson City, Tennessee

SINDHURA KOMPELLA, MD
Research Assistant, Department of Psychiatry and Behavioral Sciences, Quillen College of Medicine, East Tennessee State University, Johnson City, Tennessee

JUSTIN T. McDANIEL, PhD
Assistant Professor, Public Health and Recreation Professions, Southern Illinois University, Carbondale, Illinois

RICHARD L. SOWELL, PhD, RN, FAAN
Professor of Nursing, Research and Development Coordinator, Academy of Inclusive Learning and Social Growth, WellStar College of Health and Human Services, Kennesaw State University, Kennesaw, Georgia

TERESA M. STEPHENS, PhD, MSN, RN, CNE
Associate Professor, College of Nursing, Medical University of South Carolina, Charleston, South Carolina

KATE HENDRICKS THOMAS, PhD, MCHES
Assistant Professor of Health Sciences, Public Health Program Director, Charleston Southern University, College of Health Sciences, Charleston, South Carolina

ROXANNE F. UNDERWOOD, FNP-BC
Infectious Diseases, Quillen College of Medicine, East Tennessee State University, HIV Center of Excellence, Johnson City, Tennessee

Contents

Preface: Positive Living with Human Immunodeficiency Virus/Acquired Immunodeficiency Syndrome   xi

Kenneth D. Phillips

Exercise and Positive Living in Human Immunodeficiency Virus/AIDS   1

Jason R. Jaggers

> Evidence would suggest that regardless of disease status, people living with human immunodeficiency virus (HIV)/AIDS can obtain similar health benefits from routine physical activity reported within general populations. Research has shown significant improvements among psychological and physiologic variables within the first 5 to 6 weeks of beginning a routine physical activity program. Daily activity has shown promising results in other clinical populations, but there is still a paucity of research that limits evidence among the HIV population. Additional research is needed to examine the long-term benefits of physical activity and to discover more practical ways to achieve this lifestyle change.

Nutritional Issues and Positive Living in Human Immunodeficiency Virus/AIDS   13

William Andrew Clark and Eileen M. Cress

> Nutritional counseling has been shown to improve dietary intake in individuals with human immunodeficiency virus (HIV)/AIDS. Registered dietitians/nutritionists can individualize diet interventions to optimize effectiveness in treating metabolic consequences of the HIV infection or highly active antiretroviral therapy. Nutrition management for individuals infected with HIV can be helpful in maintaining lean body weight, combating oxidative stress, reducing complications from hyperglycemia and hyperlipidemia, and managing gastrointestinal function. Consideration should be given to including the expertise of a registered dietitian/nutritionist.

The Role of Faith-Based Organizations in the Education, Support, and Services for Persons Living with Human Immunodeficiency Virus/Acquired Immunodeficiency Syndrome   25

Teresa M. Stephens

> Faith-based organizations are in a unique position to provide resilience-enhancing efforts for persons living with human immunodeficiency virus/AIDS. Many persons living with human immunodeficiency virus/AIDS report having a strong faith or religious affiliation, with a large percentage attending church services on a regular basis. Faith-based organizations can use these factors to reach out to these individuals and effectively promote health, well-being, education, and support. Faith-based organizations can contribute to the reduction of stigma and isolation for persons living with human immunodeficiency virus/AIDS.

Mindful Living with Human Immunodeficiency Virus and AIDS: Behavioral Medicine for Patient Resilience and Improved Screening Practices   35

Kate Hendricks Thomas, Justin T. McDaniel, Aaron J. Diehr, and Kyleanne Hunter

Complementary techniques are useful in treating adverse symptoms of human immunodeficiency virus (HIV) and AIDS and in preventing disease spread by encouraging screening. This study indicates that HIV diagnosis rates are higher in states where behavioral medicine is practiced; participation in such activities may influence the extent to which someone might closely monitor personal health. A strong evidence base exists for the recommendation of mindfulness practices that improve rates of primary preventive practices and self-reported quality of life for participants living with chronic conditions such as HIV and AIDS. Access to such programs is an area for future research and practice.

Promoting Cardiovascular Health in Patients Living with Human Immunodeficiency Virus/Acquired Immunodeficiency Syndrome   47

Robin Harris

Patients living with human immunodeficiency virus/acquired immunodeficiency syndrome (PLWHA) are at an increased risk of cardiovascular disease because of advances in human immunodeficiency virus/acquired immunodeficiency syndrome treatment and increased life expectancy. Cardiovascular health promotion in PLWHA includes strategies for risk factor reduction, disease prevention, early detection, and treatment of cardiovascular disease.

Substance Use Disorders in People Living with Human Immunodeficiency Virus/AIDS   57

Priyanka Amin and Antoine Douaihy

Persons living with human immunodeficiency virus (HIV)/AIDS have a substantial burden of co-occurring substance use disorders (SUDs); untreated alcohol and drug use disorders among people living with HIV/AIDS contribute to worse HIV care outcomes. SUDs are associated with key health behaviors and outcomes, including delays in seeking medical care, poor engagement in treatment, reduced adherence to medical treatment and antiretroviral therapy, immunosuppression, increased HIV transmission through risky sexual behaviors, and increased burdens on health care systems. HIV infection comorbid with SUD and a psychiatric disorder is a clinically challenging condition creating a complex set of medical and psychosocial challenges.

Best Practices and Self-Care to Support Women in Living Well with Human Immunodeficiency Virus/AIDS   67

Melinda Ann Bogardus

Women accounted for 20% of the cumulative AIDS cases in the United States as of 2015. Although their incidence of human immunodeficiency virus (HIV) has declined in recent years, the rates of new infections and AIDS diagnoses for women of color have remained high. Women with HIV tend to be more vulnerable than men with this disease. They are more likely to be poor, uninsured, depressed, and homeless; to have experienced interpersonal violence; and to be caregivers. Attention to psychosocial needs and building trust are fundamental to engaging HIV-positive women in care and helping them attain optimal health.

Management of Coinfections in Patients with Human Immunodeficiency Virus   83

Sabra S. Custer

Many persons living with HIV use antiretrovirals for a long period of time to maintain suppression of human immunodeficiency virus (HIV) and in addition are coinfected with tuberculosis, hepatitis B, or hepatitis C. These coinfections can be successfully treated or managed alongside HIV infection. Clinicians should follow practice guidelines to appropriately screen patients with HIV for these coinfections and initiate treatment when necessary. The most significant concern when treating any of these coinfections is to avoid drug-drug interactions with the patient's antiretrovirals. Several excellent practice guidelines exist for the treatment of these common HIV coinfections.

A Therapeutic Perspective of Living with Human Immunodeficiency Virus/AIDS in 2017   97

David B. Cluck and Roxanne F. Underwood

Patients with human immunodeficiency virus (HIV)/AIDS live a far different life today compared with those who were infected in the 1980s and 1990s. Antiretroviral therapy has evolved from a once poorly tolerated, heavy pill burden to the availability of many once-daily single-tablet regimens. The improvements in therapy have necessitated the need to be cognizant of comorbidities as well as drug-drug interactions. Despite the tremendous advances in therapy, newer therapies are in the pipeline and continue to emerge, making care for patients burdened by HIV perhaps easier than it has ever been.

Stigma and Discrimination: Threats to Living Positively with Human Immunodeficiency Virus   111

Richard L. Sowell

Antiretroviral therapy and care advances have resulted in people with human immunodeficiency virus (HIV) living longer and enjoying a higher level of physical well-being. Despite such advances, individuals with HIV continue to confront challenges to living positively, including facing the secondary epidemic of stigma and discrimination. Following is a historical overview of the concept of stigma and an exploration of the causes and consequences of multilevel stigma for individuals with HIV. Strategies used by individuals and societies to manage stigma and avoid negative experiences also are examined.

End-of-Life Care and Bereavement Issues in Human Immunodeficiency Virus–AIDS   123

Karl Goodkin, Sindhura Kompella, and Steven F. Kendell

This review article addresses end-of-life care issues characterizing human immunodeficiency virus progression by delineating associated stages of medical and nursing care. The initial progression from primary medical and nursing care aimed at functional cure to palliative care is discussed. This transition is considered in accord with the major symptoms experienced, including fatigue, pain, insomnia, decreased libido, hypogonadism, memory, and concentration, depression, and distorted body image. From the stage of palliative care, progression is delineated onward through the stages of hospice care, death and dying, and the subsequent bereavement process.

NURSING CLINICS OF NORTH AMERICA

FORTHCOMING ISSUES

June 2018
Women's Health Across the Lifespan
Alice L. March, *Editor*

September 2018
Syndromes in Organ Failure
Benjamin A. Smallheer, *Editor*

December 2018
Nephrology
Deborah Ellison and Chita Farrar, *Editors*

RECENT ISSUES

December 2017
Glucose Regulation
Celia Levesque, *Editor*

September 2017
Geriatric Syndromes
Sally Miller and Jennifer Kim, *Editors*

June 2017
Fluids and Electrolytes
Joshua Squiers, *Editor*

THE CLINICS ARE AVAILABLE ONLINE!
Access your subscription at:
www.theclinics.com

NURSING CLINICS OF NORTH AMERICA

FORTHCOMING ISSUES

June 2018
Women's Health Across the Lifespan
Alice L. March, Editor

September 2018
Syndromes in Organ Failure
Benjamin A. Smallheer, Editor

December 2018
Nephrology
Deborah Ellison and Chris Ferral, Editors

RECENT ISSUES

December 2017
Glucose Regulation
Celia Levesque, Editor

September 2017
Geriatric Syndromes
Sally Miller and Jennifer Kim, Editors

June 2017
Fluids and Electrolytes
Joshua Squiers, Editor

Preface
Positive Living with Human Immunodeficiency Virus/Acquired Immunodeficiency Syndrome

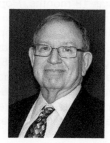

Kenneth D. Phillips, PhD, RN
Editor

Each morning we are born again—what we do today is what matters
—Buddha

I remember where I was and what I was doing when I first heard about AIDS. It was July 3, 1981. I was working as a traveling nurse, and I was enjoying a day off from my job as a staff nurse in a 12-bed intensive care unit. As I was watching CNN and drinking a cup of coffee, a brief report about a rare pneumonia in young gay men caught my attention.

After my contract as a traveling nurse ended, I returned to my home in Tennessee and to a job in a Coronary Care Unit. This was a job that fulfilled me and led me on to other educational pursuits. It was not long after I returned to Tennessee when one of my friends contacted me and told me that he had AIDS, which manifested itself as the "wasting syndrome" and Kaposi sarcoma, an opportunistic malignancy.

Sometime later, Joseph (pseudonym) asked me to come to his home and told me that he was considering assisted suicide. He introduced me to the Hemlock Society USA, a national right-to-die organization that was founded in 1980. As he made both of us a cup of tea, he was crying uncontrollably and told me he wanted to end his suffering. I let him talk, and I listened carefully as we drank the tea. I invited him to go to lunch with me, and we continued to talk. As I took him to his home, he reiterated his desire to end his life. As we parted, I asked him to call me before he took any action regarding his life, because I did not want him to die alone. That time never came, and his life ended without assisted suicide.

There was little hope in the 1980s for people who were living with human immunodeficiency virus (HIV) infection. The Centers for Disease Control and Prevention published an article on June 5, 1981 in the *Morbidity and Mortality Weekly Report*

Nurs Clin N Am 53 (2018) xi–xiii
https://doi.org/10.1016/j.cnur.2017.12.001
0029-6465/18/© 2017 Published by Elsevier Inc.

concerning five young, previously healthy gay men in Los Angeles who had come down with a rare lung infection known as *Pneumocystis carinii* pneumonia.[1] On July 3, 1981, the *New York Times* published an article titled, "Rare Cancer Seen in 41 Homosexuals."[2] This very aggressive type of cancer, Kaposi sarcoma, was known to the medical community before AIDS was recognized because it had been seen in persons who were severely immunocompromised for reasons other than AIDS. At the end of 1981, all of the first 270 AIDS cases were among gay men and 121 of them died during that year. There were no tests, treatments, or vaccines for this fatal illness. In fact, even the cause of AIDS was unknown. The average life expectancy after receiving an AIDS diagnosis was 18 months. *Hope seemed futile that year.*

It has been 36 years since HIV/AIDS was first recognized. In that 36 years, hope has slowly increased that HIV/AIDS would be conquered. It took three years from the first cases of HIV/AIDS to identify the etiologic agent. In 1983, Dr Françoise Barré-Sinnousi and her colleagues at the Pasteur Institute in France discovered a virus that they identified as a potential cause of AIDS.[3] In 1984, Dr Robert Gallo and his colleagues at the National Cancer Institute discovered a retrovirus they called the HTLV-III, which was confirmed as the etiologic agent of HIV infection.[4]

Screening and diagnostic tests for HIV infection started to become available. The first antibody test, the enzyme-linked immunosorbent assay (ELISA), was licensed by the US Food and Drug Administration in 1985. This test was highly specific, making it a good screening test. After two positive ELISA tests, the Western blot assay was used to confirm diagnosis. A drawback of the antibody tests was that it took up to 12 weeks after exposure to HIV for antibodies to appear in the blood. Antigen tests, such as polymerase chain reaction that detected HIV-1 RNA antigens, became available that significantly reduced the amount of time from exposure to diagnosis. Self-administered antibody rapid tests became available that allowed men and women to test for HIV antibodies in the privacy of their own homes. Earlier diagnosis has made earlier treatment possible.

The HIV replication cycle has been elucidated. Knowing the stages of replication has facilitated the development of six classes of antiretroviral drugs used to treat HIV infections. In those six classes, there are nearly 30 agents that alter one or more stages of the replication cycle. In the earlier days, some HIV-infected gay carried timers to remind them of the numerous pills and doses that were needed to help them combat their illness. Now, antiretroviral doses in some cases have been reduced to as little as one pill, which is taken only one time a day.

As of yet, there is still no effective vaccine to prevent the transmission of HIV infection. Much work is still being done to develop that effective vaccine. Unfortunately, the rapid rate of mutation of the virus has slowed that progress.

Today, there is great hope for those who are living with HIV/AIDS. Earlier diagnosis, effective antiretroviral therapy, and effective treatment for opportunistic infections and malignancies have greatly improved life expectancy of persons living with HIV/AIDS (PLWHA). These measures have lengthened life expectancy for PLWHA. More people are living to age 50 and beyond.[5] In this special issue of *Nursing Clinics of North America*, we suggest that by focusing on positive living with HIV infection it may even further lengthen life expectancy. Best practices and self-care strategies for women who are living with HIV infection are ways to improve their quality of life. In addition to pharmacologic management of HIV infection, authors in this special issue have proposed exercise, nutrition, the management of coinfections, promotion of faith and resiliency, mindfulness living, promotion of cardiovascular health, combating substance abuse, and dealing with stigma and end-of-life issues as ways to live more positive lives with HIV infection.

Kenneth D. Phillips, PhD, RN
College of Nursing
East Tennessee State University
Johnson City, TN 37614, USA

E-mail address:
phillipskd@mail.etsu.edu

REFERENCES

1. Centers for Disease Control. Pneumocystis pneumonia--Los Angeles. MMWR Morb Mortal Wkly Rep 1981;30(21):250–2.
2. Altman LK. Rare cancer seen in 41 homosexuals. The New York Times 1981. Available at: http://www.nytimes.com/1981/07/03/us/rare-cancer-seen-in-41-homosexuals.html. Accessed December 13, 2017.
3. Barré-Sinoussi F, Chermann JC, Rey F, et al. Isolation of a T-lymphotropic retrovirus from a patient at risk for acquired immune deficiency syndrome (AIDS). Science 1983;220(4599):868–71.
4. Gallo RC, Salahuddin SZ, Popovic M, et al. Frequent detection and isolation of cytopathic retroviruses (HTLV-III) from patients with AIDS and at risk for AIDS. Science 1984;224(4648):500–3.
5. Teeraananchai S, Kerr SJ, Amin J, et al. Life expectancy of HIV-positive people after starting combination antiretroviral therapy: a meta-analysis. HIV Med 2017;18:256–66.

Exercise and Positive Living in Human Immunodeficiency Virus/AIDS

Jason R. Jaggers, PhD

KEYWORDS

• Physical activity • Fitness • Exercise • Stress • HIV

KEY POINTS

- Exercise can be both safe and beneficial for this clinical population, making it imperative to determine successful motivational and behavioral-changing interventions aimed at increasing physical activity.
- Routine physical activity has shown to reduce daily stress and circulating cortisol in as few as 3 weeks among people living with human immunodeficiency virus (HIV)/AIDS.
- Individuals do not necessarily have to work at a vigorous intensity level to achieve significant health benefits as long as they stay consistent with their exercise plan.
- The important takeaway regarding exercise and the immune system is that research among HIV populations has demonstrated that exercise performed at low, moderate, or high intensity does not negatively impact immune function or disease progression in HIV-infected individuals.

INTRODUCTION

It was not until long after Plato once said "Lack of activity destroys the good condition of every human being, while movement and methodical physical exercise save it and preserve it" that exercise science and the field of epidemiology began getting the world's attention regarding the health benefits of physical activity and its overall importance to stay mobile. Even though it may have taken more than 3000 years for most of the world to take these words seriously, scientific discoveries on the topic have exploded since the mid-1900s. With regard to the relevance on public health, the biggest strides have been made with the general population in relationship to risk of chronic diseases, as well as some clinical research in areas like cardiovascular

Conflicts of Interest: The author of this article has no financial disclosures or conflicts of interest to disclose.
Department of Health and Sport Sciences, University of Louisville, 2100 South Floyd Street SAC East 104, Louisville, KY 40208, USA
E-mail address: Jason.jaggers@louisville.edu

disease and rehabilitative physical therapy following injury. The irony of this research with clinical populations is that had they been physically active beforehand, that injury or heart attack may have been prevented in the first place. However, not all clinical populations are diagnosed with a disease that could have been prevented by physical activity, diet, or other healthy lifestyle factors.

Some chronic conditions, like viral infections, are facing a multitude of problems from a diagnosis that could have occurred no matter how physically fit or health conscious the individual was 99% of their lives. One such condition, such as human immunodeficiency virus (HIV), is accompanied by a lifetime of medications known to disrupt metabolic processes, creating a metabolic syndrome–like condition. Many of these metabolic disruptions are known to increase one's risk for chronic diseases but evidence would suggest they could possibly be offset by maintaining an active lifestyle. With weekly exercise regimens prescribed as a form of complementary treatment, this in turn could help reduce the risk of chronic disease and mortality for people living with HIV/AIDS (PLWHA). Although we have strong evidence demonstrating the clear benefits of exercise in the general population, whether the same level of benefit is possible among individuals living with HIV remains less clear. What we do know with regard to the benefits of exercise for PLWHA is discussed in this review of the literature from research conducted since the beginning of the epidemic. This in turn will lead into a brief discussion about psychoneuroimmunology (PNI) theory and the interconnections of the mind, body, and one's self.

EXERCISE AND HUMAN IMMUNODEFICIENCY VIRUS: THE KNOWN BENEFITS

Exercise is defined as a "type of physical activity consisting of planned, structured, and repetitive bodily movement done to improve and/or maintain one of more components of physical fitness."[1] It is important to note that "exercise" by definition does not need to begin immediately for PLWHA to gain mental and physical health benefits. Recent evidence would suggest simply an increase in daily physical activity by adding more steps per day can have a significant impact on waist circumference and activities of daily living.[2] Short-term goals, like an increase in daily steps, is a great way to begin implementing positive habits that will improve health and quality of life without the need for 150 minutes of moderate-intensity exercise every week. Obviously, that would be the ultimate long-term goal for every person wanting to live a longer, healthier life, but for someone who has been primarily sedentary for a prolonged period, like most people with HIV, starting with a more realistic approach of just walking more could prove beneficial. What makes this of even greater importance is the known associations between cardiorespiratory fitness (CRF) and all-cause mortality. Research has suggested individuals with lower CRF are at an increased risk for cardiovascular disease (CVD), stroke, hypertension, diabetes, cancer, all-cause mortality, and many more chronic conditions.[3–5]

People of all ages infected with HIV have abnormally low levels of CRF.[6–12] These reductions have been attributed to sedentary behavior and lifestyle habits. Further, PLWHA often exhibit a maximal Vo_2 of 24% to 44% below their age-predicted normal values.[6–12] CRF, as determined by maximal Vo_2, is a powerful predictor of all-cause and CVD mortality and of type 2 diabetes mellitus.[3,5,13,14] Evidence from clinical exercise investigations would suggest that a moderate-intensity physical activity regimen can produce adaptations leading to an increased CRF.[6,13–15] These investigations are severely limited considering they range from only 6 to 12 weeks, use various training protocols rarely mimicking that of others, and most importantly there is a lack of larger trials or even longitudinal investigations that incorporate physical activity as a regular part of their follow-up periods. Some of these are discussed further in greater detail, but for a summary of these studies and their findings, see **Table 1**.

Although limited scientific information exists, the effects of routine exercise at moderate intensities have shown health benefits among PLWHA as an alternative form of treatment. Studies have shown significant improvements in CRF, muscular strength, body composition, and mental health after 6 weeks of moderate-intensity aerobic training when completed 2 to 3 days per week.[16–18] Further, there have not been any detriments to immunologic status or increases in disease progression due to routine exercise reported within the literature. Benefits of a structured exercise prescription among PLWHA include increases in muscle mass and strength, decreased fat mass and waist circumference, possible improvements in circulating lipids (triglycerides, total cholesterol, low-density lipoprotein), decreases in self-reported depression and anxiety, enhanced psychological well-being, increased quality of life, and increases in CRF.[16–18] Many of these health benefits are known to reduce risk of CVD, metabolic abnormalities, psychological disturbance, and all-cause mortality in clinical and general populations.[13,14,19] In return, people will typically also have an increased sense of well-being, improved outlook on life, and alleviate their levels of stress, which is critical for PLWHA due to the negative perceptions often experienced when learning of their diagnosis.

The stigmatization in which society has placed on persons infected with HIV, along with the personal perceived stressors, has resulted in numerous psychological disturbances experienced immediately on learning of a positive HIV diagnosis. Rates of anxiety and depressive symptoms among this population remain consistently high regardless of treatment, patient demographics, or socioeconomic status. A coping mechanism proven to be successful time and time again in all facets of research is social support, especially in relationship to stress reduction, managing a chronic condition, and even adhering to an exercise or diet regimen. In essence, this makes social support, interpersonal relationships, and one's sense of human connections all potential mediators to a magnitude of issues. Although often studied separately, when combining the fields of psychology and physiology, the outcomes can be quite fascinating. The idea that our thoughts can wreak havoc on our internal systems is relatively

Table 1
Exercise and positive health benefits

Body System	Response to Exercise
Psychological	• ↓ depressive symptoms[2,20,23] • ↓ anxiety[21,22] • ↑ mood state[2,20–22,34]

Physiologic	• ↑ Vo$_2$ peak[6,9,16,22,25,35]
	  ○ Significant increases between 2.40 and 3.71 mL/kg/min[18]
	• ↑ Strength[28,35,36]
	• ↓ Fat mass and waist circumference[2,20,28,37,38]
	• ↓ Cortisol[2,28]
	• ↑ GH, IL-6, and sTNFrII[28]
	  ○ Acute increase post exercise
	• Blood lipids[37,39]
	  ○ Conflicting results

Immunologic	• ↑ CD4+[10,40] • No change in CD4+[12,22,25,35,41]

Abbreviations: GH, growth hormone; IL-6, interleukin-6; sTNFrII, tumor necrosis factor. ↑ indicates increased; ↓ indicates decreased.

new in both fields, but one that must be taken into account when improving the health of PLWHA.

Psychological Improvements

Early investigations conducted before antiretroviral therapy (ART) compared the effects of aerobic exercise on psychological components, such as depression and anxiety. Eight weeks of moderate-intensity aerobic exercise completed twice a week for 60 minutes has shown significant reductions in anxiety and depression.[2,20–23] Other investigators reported significant improvements after only 5 weeks of aerobic exercise.[21] Men who exercised for 45 minutes a day, 3 days a week, reduced anxiety and depression on learning of their seropositive status.[21] Limitations to these early investigations are evident because they were conducted before current ART regimens during a time when symptoms were specific to viral progression and not treatment. Further, most study demographics also consisted of middle class gay men. Due to the shift in patient demographics and treatments, those findings lack generalizability with today's seropositive populations. However, more recent investigations have begun showing promising results, suggesting exercise as a viable coping mechanism when battling depression and anxiety.

Another important factor to consider when comparing findings is that aerobic and resistance training both have very different physiologic adaptations, so it would seem plausible to expect added psychological benefits when the 2 are combined during routine exercise training. However, a major limitation with previous investigations among clinical and healthy populations is that they incorporated only one type of exercise training, but not both. There have been only a few investigations that compared the differences between aerobic and resistance training on psychological health by randomizing participants into an aerobic or resistance training program, but failed to include a group that combined the two. These studies reported similar psychological improvements between groups.

Results of these investigations demonstrate that PLWHA are able to obtain beneficial results among self-reported psychological disturbances, primarily total mood state and depression, through various forms of routine exercise in as little as 5 to 6 weeks. Stronger evidence supports aerobic as the preferred type of exercise, but specific dosages regarding time and intensity have yet to be identified due to a lack of homogeneity among study methods. However, as more research uses a combination of aerobic and resistance training, we could begin to see similar results with additional improvements in body composition and strength. These interventions did not, however, elicit any changes to self-reported frequency of symptoms, symptom distress, or fatigue associated with HIV and/or treatment. Even though there were not any changes in symptomatology or its related distress, PLWHA were still able to improve their mood state and reduce depression. This would suggest that resistance and/or aerobic training can enhance psychological well-being independent of symptomatology.

Physiologic Improvements

In addition to positive psychological effects, there is also strong evidence indicating the physiologic improvements across clinical measurements of health, such as body mass index (BMI), waist circumference, blood lipids, strength, and CRF (among others). Similar to the psychological benefits previously explained, some of these were noticeable within 6 weeks. However, what is interesting to note is that stronger gains were observed following longer durations independent of intensity, suggesting individuals do not necessarily have to work at a vigorous intensity level as long as they stay consistent with their exercise plan. A 24-week exercise intervention using 2 levels of intensity (medium or high) found both intensities yielded significant improvements in CRF and reduced perceived stress. The medium-intensity group exercised 3 times a week at 50% to 60% of their Vo_{2max} for 40 minutes and the high-intensity group exercised 3 times a week at 75% to 85% of their Vo_{2max} for 24 minutes. A major limitation to that study, however, was the high attrition rate of 76%, which was possibly due to the long duration or intensity of the study.[9] In a similar clinical trial, participants were randomized into either a high-intensity or moderate-intensity aerobic exercise group and exercised for a total of 30 minutes, 3 days a week for 12 weeks. Findings showed a significant improvement in functional capacity, measured by time to fatigue, in both groups.[24]

Even interventions consisting of low-intensity aerobic exercise, but with a longer duration of 16 weeks, have also shown significant improvements among CRF and high-density lipoprotein cholesterol when compared with a control group. Further, there were significant decreases in total abdominal adipose tissue, total cholesterol, and circulating triglycerides.[25] Similar results have been reported by other researchers who have found significant increases in CRF, oxygen pulse, and maximum tidal volume, but not blood lipids. In addition, aerobic exercise has demonstrated decreases in BMI, waist-to-hip ratio, body density, and body fat after a 12-week moderate-intensity aerobic exercise intervention.[26]

The reported findings would, thus, indicate that PLWHA are able to elicit significant health improvements when following a prescribed exercise routine lasting 5 weeks or longer. These effects have been observed regardless of the exercise intensity, participant disease status, and/or current antiretroviral treatment.[16–18] Current data seem to suggest that any amount of routine physical activity will elicit health gains among PLWHA, but, similar to the general population, more health gains can be achieved with higher intensities and/or longer durations. However, as noted previously, due to the deconditioned state of most sedentary individuals, larger gains can be made in a shorter period without doing as much. Studies have shown that just making slight adjustments to increase activity habits has had positive benefits on various types of stressors and health variables.

With regard to the physiologic effects from chronic stress, it is well known that excess cortisol secretion can negatively affect multiple processes within the body. Even though this stress hormone can be secreted due to internal stressors or a perceived stressor from the surrounding environment, individuals living with HIV will often amplify the stress response from the moment of diagnosis. Evidence has also demonstrated its negative effects on immunity and overall health.[21,27] For example, the acute stress response has been shown to be associated with enhanced immunity, whereas chronic stressors are known to suppress immune function. Although exercise-related research and cortisol secretion in patients with HIV is lacking, the few studies that have measured the physiologic stressor cortisol indicates significant reductions in the levels of secretion after just a few weeks of combination exercise.[20,28] What is more encouraging is that the evidence would suggest reductions by nearly half of circulating morning cortisol levels can be achieved without necessarily having to meet the minimum recommendations of daily exercise.

One investigation showed that the individuals in the exercise group significantly decreased morning salivary cortisol by 49% when compared with the control group (which showed no change). Exercisers completed only a total of 90 minutes of aerobic activity per week combined with 2 days of moderate-intensity resistance training. To our knowledge, this was the first clinical exercise study to report area under the curve measures of waking cortisol in HIV-positive persons before and after an exercise intervention.[20] This reduction in salivary cortisol may have been mediated by the reduction of depressive symptoms also observed in the same study. Others have identified hyperactivity of the hypothalamic-pituitary-adrenal axis in depressed individuals during stressful periods, often resulting in elevated circulating cortisol. Exercise effectively reduces circulating levels of cortisol and depressive symptoms in a wide range of populations. In the study just described, all but 1 of the participants who decreased salivary cortisol at wake also decreased their total Profile of Mood States and depression scores.[20] However, much more research on physiologic and psychological stress in relationship to exercise is needed to further support these findings. The ability to lessen the degree of chronic stress experienced on a daily basis should lead to improvements in immunity and thus overall health.

Effects of Exercise on Immunologic Variables

In addition to their findings on physiologic and psychological variables, no significant changes in CD4+ count have been reported in both the high-intensity and moderate-intensity groups.[10,18,22,23,29] Further, there have been no significant changes from baseline reported in CD4+ cell count, CD8+ cell count, leukocytes, or lymphocytes following moderate or high-intensity exercise. Recently it was shown that patients with dyslipidemia and lipodystrophy had no significant changes in immunologic variables after completing 12 weeks of moderate-intensity aerobic exercise as well. These results are promising; however, more immunologic improvements may be observed with the success of prolonged stress reduction either in the form of psychological distress or the stress hormone cortisol.

Chronic stress is believed to enhance the antibody-mediated humeral response, while suppressing other areas of immunity. In addition to immunosuppressive effects, chronic stress is known to also increase systemic inflammation. Research has demonstrated that an increase in circulating biomarkers of inflammation (C-reactive protein, interleukin [IL]-6) results from a chronic state of stress.[30] These biomarkers are also clearly established to increase the risk of CVD and infectious diseases among general populations. Evidence exists supporting the idea that the immune responses occur both from psychosocial factors as well as physical harm. There are also published findings with supporting evidence to suggest self-reported perceived stress, anxiety, depression, and anger are associated with higher proinflammatory cytokine levels of IL-1, IL-6, and tumor necrosis factor alpha.[31] Even more alarming is the known association that these cytokines can facilitate viral replication.

The important takeaway regarding exercise and the immune system is that research among PLWHA has demonstrated that aerobic exercise performed at low, moderate, or high intensity does not negatively impact immune function or disease progression in HIV-infected individuals. This suggests that aerobic exercise can be both beneficial and safe for this clinical population. However, it is recommended that if aerobic exercise is to be performed by this population, that they do so at a low-intensity or moderate-intensity level, as data are lacking to draw the conclusion that a high-intensity aerobic regimen will not have a negative impact on overall health or quality of life in this population.[1,6,17]

Psycho-Physio Connections and Immunity

The study of neural, endocrine, and immune system interactions known as PNI theory is believed to elicit communication between the neuroendocrine and immune systems. This relationship can be explained by PNI involving the following 5 systems: (1) hypothalamic, pituitary, and adrenal hormones; (2) cytokines; (3) neuropeptides; (4) neurotransmitters; and (5) the sympathetic nervous system. Considering the connected networks among these systems as well as the cascading events involved when activated, the idea of a behavioral and biological mechanism linking psychosocial factors, health, and disease is the primary emphasis of PNI. This concept cannot be explained in a matter of a few paragraphs so a model representing the interconnections of each component is shown in **Fig. 1**.

What is more important is that health care professionals should look to apply some of the theoretic framework behind PNI to any human health condition through stress reduction techniques. This in turn can help identify patterns, processes, and consequences of stress as it relates to health and/or disease dynamics while strengthening our understanding of psychosocial and physiologic factors influencing immunity. An emerging topic in current health care literature is mindful meditation, which can be applied to any population experiencing high stress and/or poor health. This and many other stress reduction techniques go hand in hand with improving long-term care and prognosis. What is even more interesting is the linkage between exercise adaptations for each of the 5 components of PNI.

SUMMARY

Aerobic and resistance exercise both have multiple physiologic benefits (ie, increased cardiorespiratory fitness and strength, improvements in body composition, enhanced functional ability) that in turn lead to improvements in psychological health, such as improved self-esteem and overall quality of life. Multiple studies have continuously shown increased cardiorespiratory fitness, improved body composition, and increased muscular strength, which has continued to be supported in recent publications. Additional psychological benefits have also been observed independent of improved physiologic health.

Evidence would suggest that PLWHA, regardless of disease status, can obtain similar short-term health benefits from routine physical activity reported within general populations. Research has shown significant improvements among psychological and physiologic variables after moderate levels of routine exercise within the first 5 to 6 weeks of beginning a routine physical activity program. It is also clear that across various populations, routine moderate-intensity physical activity reduces the risk of chronic disease and that many of these conditions have been established as major causes of morbidity and mortality among PLWHA. With clear evidence showing that physical activity can be both safe and beneficial for this clinical population, it is imperative we now determine successful motivational and behavioral-changing interventions aimed at increasing physical activity and other positive health habits, such as smoking cessation, diet, and stress reduction, among others.

To improve health outcomes of PLWHA and reduce health disparities, it is important that health and wellness professionals understand that like most health habits, physical activity behavior is influenced by individual (eg, knowledge, attitudes, skills), interpersonal (eg, family, friends), organizational (eg, workplace, clinics), and community factors (eg, built or natural physical environment).[32] Further, it is critical to provide excellent resources for proper health education and local connections for social support for PLWHA to incorporate daily exercise into their lives. Health and fitness professionals also need to consider innovative health programming options for those who have limited means to transportation, finances, and/or access to facilities.

Recommendations for Exercise

Current exercise training recommendations as described in the American College of Sports Medicine's *Exercise Management for Persons with Chronic Disease and*

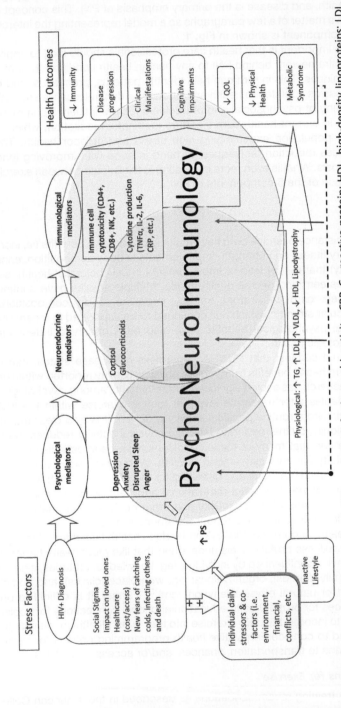

Fig. 1. PNI-based model of stress-related effects on HIV infection and inactivity. CRP, C - reactive protein; HDL, high-density lipoproteins; LDL, low-density lipoproteins; NE, norepinephrine; NK, natural killer cells; PS, perceived stress; QOL, quality of life; TG, triglycerides; TNFα, tumor necrosis factor alpha; VLDL, very low density lipoprotein. ↑ indicates increased; ↓ indicates decreased; + indicates "adds to".

Disabilities (4th edition) for PLWHA suggest a moderate-intensity aerobic and resistance training regimen similar to recommendations for the general population.[1] This includes accumulating a total of 150 minutes of moderate-intensity physical activity a week, as well as 2 days of full-body resistance training at approximately 60% of 1 repetition maximum. Although this goal is perfectly safe for anyone without underlying heart problems, it may not necessarily be realistic for someone living with HIV starting a program. As previously discussed, anyone going from a primarily sedentary lifestyle to one of increased activity will see improvements just by moving more. However, there are still increased risks involved that cannot be ignored, more so as a precautionary measure to avoid undue harm onto individuals when their full health history is unknown.

Regardless of disease status, it is strongly recommended that anyone living with HIV or AIDS receive medical clearance from their primary health care provider before beginning an exercise program. Responses and adaptations to exercise training will vary depending on current fitness level, disease status, and whether or not that patient is currently on an ART regimen. Asymptomatic individuals generally respond in a manner similar to someone without HIV of the same body size, age, and gender. However, some may be more deconditioned due to psychological disturbances commonly associated with daily sedentary behavior, such as depression or anxiety, among others.

Daily activity has shown promising results in other clinical populations, but there is still a paucity of research that limits evidence among the HIV population. Additional research is needed to not only test the hypothesis that long-term changes in physical activity behaviors would improve quality of life by helping self-manage the illness, but also to discover more cost-effective and practical ways to achieve this lifestyle change.[32,33]

REFERENCES

1. Moore G, Durstine JL, Painter P. Medicine ACoS. ACSM's exercise management for persons with chronic diseases and disabilities, 4E. Human Kinetics; 2016.
2. Jaggers JR, Sneed JM, Lobelo RF, et al. Results of a nine month home-based physical activity intervention for people living with HIV. Int J Clin Trials 2016; 3(3):106–19.
3. Blair SN, Kampert JB, Kohl HW, et al. Influences of cardiorespiratory fitness and other precursors on cardiovascular disease and all-cause mortality in men and women. Jama 1996;276(3):205–10.
4. Haskell WL, Lee IM, Pate RR, et al. Physical activity and public health: updated recommendation for adults from the American College of Sports Medicine and the American Heart Association. Circulation 2007;116(9):1081.
5. LaMonte MJ, Blair SN. Physical activity, cardiorespiratory fitness, and adiposity: contributions to disease risk. Curr Opin Clin Nutr Metab Care 2006;9(5):540–6.
6. Hand GA, Phillips KD, Dudgeon WD, et al. Moderate intensity exercise training reverses functional aerobic impairment in HIV-infected individuals. AIDS care 2008;20(9):1066–74.
7. Jaggers JR, Dudgeon W, Blair SN, et al. A home-based exercise intervention to increase physical activity among people living with HIV: study design of a randomized clinical trial. BMC Public Health 2013;13:502.
8. Johnson JE, Anders GT, Blanton HM, et al. Exercise dysfunction in patients seropositive for the human immunodeficiency virus. Am Rev Respir Dis 1990;141(3): 618–22.

9. MacArthur RD, Levine SD, Birk TJ. Supervised exercise training improves cardio-pulmonary fitness in HIV-infected persons. Med Sci Sports Exerc 1993;25(6): 684–8.

10. Perna FM, LaPerriere A, Klimas N, et al. Cardiopulmonary and CD4 cell changes in response to exercise training in early symptomatic HIV infection. Med Sci Sports Exerc 1999;31(7):973–9.

11. Pothoff G, Wassermann K, Ostmann H. Impairment of exercise capacity in various groups of HIV-infected patients. Respiration 1994;61(2):80–5.

12. Stringer WW, Berezovskaya M, O'Brien WA, et al. The effect of exercise training on aerobic fitness, immune indices, and quality of life in HIV+ patients. Med Sci Sports Exerc 1998;30(1):11–6.

13. Church TS, Blair SN, Cocreham S, et al. Effects of aerobic and resistance training on hemoglobin A1c levels in patients with type 2 diabetes: a randomized controlled trial. JAMA 2010;304(20):2253–62.

14. Katzmarzyk PT, Church TS, Blair SN. Cardiorespiratory fitness attenuates the effects of the metabolic syndrome on all-cause and cardiovascular disease mortality in men. Arch Intern Med 2004;164(10):1092–7.

15. Hand GA, Phillips KD, Sowell RL, et al. Prevalence of poor sleep quality in a HIV+ population of African Americans. J South Carolina Med Assoc 2008;(99):183–7.

16. Hand GA, Lyerly GW, Jaggers JR, et al. Impact of aerobic and resistance exercise on the health of HIV-infected persons. Am J Lifestyle Med 2009;3(6):489–99.

17. Jaggers JR, Hand GA. Health benefits of exercise for people living with HIV: a review of the literature. Am J Lifestyle Med 2016;10(3):184–92.

18. O'Brien KK, Tynan AM, Nixon SA, et al. Effectiveness of aerobic exercise for adults living with HIV: systematic review and meta-analysis using the Cochrane Collaboration protocol. BMC Infect Dis 2016;16:182.

19. Earnest CP, Johannsen NM, Swift DL, et al. Aerobic and strength training in concomitant metabolic syndrome and type 2 diabetes. Med Sci Sports Exerc 2014;46(7):1293–301.

20. Jaggers JR, Hand GA, Dudgeon WD, et al. Aerobic and resistance training improves mood state among adults living with HIV. Int J Sports Med 2015;36(2): 175–81.

21. LaPerriere A, Ironson G, Antoni MH, et al. Exercise and psychoneuroimmunology. Med Sci Sports Exerc 1994;26(2):182–90.

22. Smith BA, Neidig JL, Nickel JT, et al. Aerobic exercise: effects on parameters related to fatigue, dyspnea, weight and body composition in HIV-infected adults. AIDS 2001;15(6):693–701.

23. Neidig JL, Smith BA, Brashers DE. Aerobic exercise training for depressive symptom management in adults living with HIV infection. J Assoc Nurses AIDS Care 2003;14(2):30–40.

24. Maharaj SS, Chetty V. Rehabilitation program for the quality of life for individuals on highly active antiretroviral therapy in KwaZulu-Natal, South Africa: a short report. Int J Rehabil Res 2011;34(4):360–5.

25. Mutimura E, Crowther NJ, Cade TW, et al. Exercise training reduces central adiposity and improves metabolic indices in HAART-treated HIV-positive subjects in Rwanda: a randomized controlled trial. AIDS Res Hum Retroviruses 2008; 24(1):15–23.

26. Driscoll SD, Meininger GE, Lareau MT, et al. Effects of exercise training and metformin on body composition and cardiovascular indices in HIV-infected patients. AIDS 2004;18(3):465–73.

27. Perna FM, Schneiderman N, LaPerriere A. Psychological stress, exercise and immunity. Int J Sports Med 1997;18(Suppl 1):S78–83.
28. Dudgeon WD, Jaggers JR, Phillips KD, et al. Moderate-intensity exercise improves body composition and improves physiological markers of stress in HIV-infected men. ISRN AIDS 2012;2012:145127.
29. Terry L, Sprinz E, Stein R, et al. Exercise training in HIV-1-infected individuals with dyslipidemia and lipodystrophy. Med Sci Sports Exerc 2006;38(3):411–7.
30. Wang TD, Wang YH, Huang TS, et al. Circulating levels of markers of inflammation and endothelial activation are increased in men with chronic spinal cord injury. J Formos Med Assoc 2007;106(11):919–28.
31. Glaser R, Kiecolt-Glaser JK, Marucha PT, et al. Stress-related changes in proinflammatory cytokine production in wounds. Arch Gen Psychiatry 1999;56(5):450–6.
32. McLeroy KR, Bibeau D, Steckler A, et al. An ecological perspective on health promotion programs. Health Education Q 1988;15:351–77.
33. Sallis JF, Owen N. Ecological models of health behavior. In: Glanz K, Rimer BK, Viswanath K, editors. Health behavior: theory, research, and practice. 5th edition. San Francisco: Wiley; 2015. p. 43–64.
34. Patil R, Shimpi A, Rairikar S, et al. Effects of fitness training on physical fitness parameters and quality of life in human immunodeficiency virus-positive Indian females. Indian J Sex Transm Dis 2017;38(1):47–53.
35. Dolan SE, Frontera W, Librizzi J, et al. Effects of a supervised home-based aerobic and progressive resistance training regimen in women infected with human immunodeficiency virus: a randomized trial. Arch Intern Med 2006;166(11):1225–31.
36. Fitch K, Abbara S, Lee H, et al. Effects of lifestyle modification and metformin on atherosclerotic indices among HIV-infected patients with the metabolic syndrome. AIDS 2012;26(5):587–97.
37. Engelson ES, Agin D, Kenya S, et al. Body composition and metabolic effects of a diet and exercise weight loss regimen on obese, HIV-infected women. Metabolism 2006;55(10):1327–36.
38. Jaggers JR, Prasad VK, Dudgeon WD, et al. Associations between physical activity and sedentary time on components of metabolic syndrome among adults with HIV. AIDS Care 2014;26(11):1387–92.
39. Thoni G, Fedou C, Brun J, et al. Reduction of fat accumulation and lipid disorders by individualized light aerobic training in human immunodeficiency virus infected patients with lipodystrophy and/or dyslipidemia. Diabetes Metab 2002;28(5):397–404.
40. LaPerriere A, Klimas N, Fletcher MA, et al. Change in CD4+ cell enumeration following aerobic exercise training in HIV-1 disease: possible mechanisms and practical applications. Int J Sports Med 1997;18(Suppl 1):S56–61.
41. Terry L, Sprinz E, Ribeiro J. Moderate and high intensity exercise training in HIV-1 seropositive individuals: a randomized trial. Int J Sports Med 1999;20(02):142–6.

Nutritional Issues and Positive Living in Human Immunodeficiency Virus/AIDS

William Andrew Clark, PhD, RD[a],*, Eileen M. Cress, EdD, RD[b]

KEYWORDS

- Food safety • Hyperlipidemia • Oxidative stress • Diabetes • Antioxidant
- Malabsorption • Nutrition counseling

KEY POINTS

- Nutrition management for individuals infected with HIV can be helpful in maintaining lean body weight, combating oxidative stress, reducing complications from hyperglycemia and hyperlipidemia, and managing gastrointestinal function.
- Patients may need to be individualized to meet each individual's unique requirements.
- Consideration should be given to including the expertise of a registered dietitian/nutritionist as part of the health care team to promote wellness in the individuals infected with HIV.

INTRODUCTION

With the advent of pharmacologic protease inhibitors (PIs) and highly active antiretroviral therapy (HAART), treatment of human immunodeficiency virus (HIV)/AIDS has made significant advances with resultant increases in life expectancy[1] and well-being.[2] The disease state itself (viral load), decreases in CD4 (white blood cell, T-cells) counts, and pharmacologic treatment protocols have created several physiologic issues that can be detrimental to the patients' health in many cases; however, these conditions can be counteracted by dietary intervention. Many persons with an HIV infection and undergoing treatment with HAART still experience weight loss, hyperglycemia, oxidative stress, hyperlipidemia, gastrointestinal issues (diarrhea and malabsorption), and fat redistribution in the body. This article provides nutrition advice for individuals infected with HIV/AIDS who are receiving PI or HAART treatment, have CD4 counts more than 200 cells/μL and are in stable condition.

Disclosure: Neither author has a conflict of interest regarding this document, and they have received no financial compensation.
^a Department of Allied Health Sciences, College of Clinical and Rehabilitative Health Sciences, East Tennessee State University, PO Box 70282, Johnson City, TN 37614, USA; ^b James H. Quillen Veterans Administration Medical Center, PO Box 4000, Mountain Home, TN 37684, USA
* Corresponding author.
E-mail address: clarkw@etsu.edu

Energy Expenditure

"A sick person's nutrition is further aggravated by diarrhea, malabsorption, loss of appetite, diversion of nutrients for the immune response, and urinary nitrogen loss, all of which lead to nutrient losses and further damage to defense mechanisms. These, in turn, caused reduced dietary intake. In addition, fever increases both energy and micronutrient requirements."[3] Energy requirements are higher in asymptomatic individuals infected with HIV, with most estimates indicating a resting metabolic rate about 10% higher than that of individuals not infected, and nutrient requirements increase with the severity of the disease.[4–7] A World Health Organization report[8] suggests an increased energy requirement between 20% and 30% during periods of symptomatic disease or opportunistic infection. Weight maintenance is a primary goal for patients with HIV/AIDS. Contributing factors to weight loss include increased energy and protein needs during periods of infection; anorexia; and common side effects of malabsorption, nausea, vomiting, or diarrhea. Fat malabsorption and steroid-induced diabetes may also occur.

Powanda and Beisel[9] reported that the catabolic nature of infections can be seen with weight loss and a correlating negative nitrogen balance. They reported that, "the translocation of amino acids from muscle to liver not only leads to increased amino acid degradation and increased urinary nitrogen excretion, but also permits an increased synthesis of plasma protein, that of the acute-phase proteins,"[9] which may assist in combating the infection. Diets that meet increased nutrient requirements for both energy and protein during periods of infection seem to be able to protect against a negative nitrogen balance.[10,11] In their report on energy expenditure and wasting in individuals infected with HIV, Macallan and colleagues[12] reported that reduced energy intake and not increased energy expenditure was primarily responsible for the resulting weight loss.

Fig. 1 shows the cycle between malnutrition and infection and the resulting physiologic consequences that result from undernutrition. Even after establishment of effective HAART treatments, Mangili and associates[13] reported that "HIV-associated weight loss is common in persons with HIV infection, regardless of whether HAART is used, and that appears to have a multifactorial etiology."[13] Wilson and colleagues[14] established a linear relationship between lean body mass and health-related quality-of-life issues in men infected with HIV. Maintenance of body weight is critical to the health of patients infected with HIV but is challenged by appetite loss (infection and pharmaceutical related), nutrient malabsorption, and inadequate dietary intake. Appetite stimulants, megestrol acetate, and oxandrolone have been used successfully to increase weight gains[15] in individuals infected with HIV receiving HAART and who have weight loss greater than 5 kg. Although maintaining weight during periods when the patient is symptomatic is difficult, recovery of weight during asymptomatic periods is critical for maintaining lean body mass in individuals infected with HIV. This period of make-up weight gain after symptomatic periods is critical in maintaining the best quality of life for individuals with an HIV infection.

Increased energy and protein needs present during periods of infection, complicated by anorexia and general fatigue, and inhibit the ability to maintain weight. Addition of nutrient-dense items to foods consumed can help meet these increased needs. Protein can be enhanced by adding powdered milk, protein powders, instant breakfast, cheese, cottage cheese, puddings, Greek yogurt, peanut butter and other nuts and butters, and well-cooked eggs to foods. Calories can be enhanced through the addition of foods such as vegetable oil, sour cream, mayonnaise, whole milk (versus skim milk), nut butters, and ice cream. Nutritional

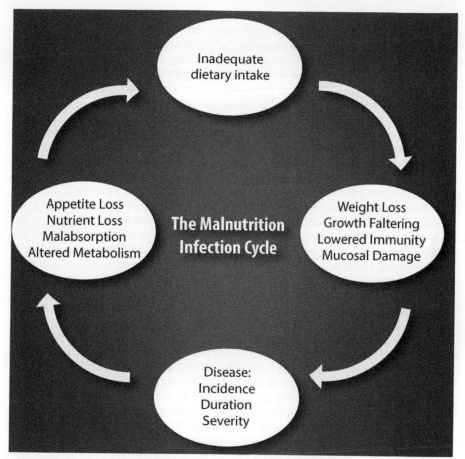

Fig. 1. The spiral of malnutrition and infection. (*From* Katona P, Katona-Apte J. The interaction between nutrition and infection. Clin Infect Dis 2008;46:1583; with permission.)

counseling can include guidelines for home-prepared supplements and meal enhancements.

When dietary intake is inadequate, oral commercial nutritional supplements and bars can be prescribed. Supplements with medium-chain fats are recommended when fat malabsorption is present. Commercial formulations are available and specialized products can be prescribed for individuals with diabetes, liver disease, or renal disease. In addition, care should be exercised because food insecurity is prevalent among patients infected with HIV, particularly women, in modern Western cultures because of diminished economic capacity and decreased physical ability, especially during symptomatic periods.[16]

Nutrient Malabsorption

Nutrient malabsorption is prevalent in many patients infected with HIV and is seen clinically through wasting (loss of lean body mass), fat malabsorption, and diarrhea. HAART has dramatically reduced the incidence of diarrhea caused by opportunistic infections (eg, *Cryptosporidium* and *Mycobacterium*); however, the incidence of diarrhea is still high.[17] In a cohort of 671 persons infected with HIV,[18] gastrointestinal dysfunction was common (>85%). Widespread malabsorption of D-xylose and borderline serum levels of vitamin B_{12} were reported. Fat malabsorption was reported in 12.8% of the cohort,[18] whereas studies with symptomatic patients with HIV showed fat malabsorption ranging from 49% to 84%.[19,20] Poles and colleagues[17] hypothesized that the high incidence of fat malabsorption (41%) seen in non-HAART and HAART-treated patients may be caused by small bowel bacterial overgrowth; however, other researchers have not seen small bowel bacterial overgrowth in similar HIV populations.[21]

Brenchley and Douek,[22] in their review article, state that early in HIV infection there is an increased level of inflammation and decreased levels of mucosal repair and regeneration and that the infection decreases the level of lamina propria CD4 T cells even when subjected to HAART treatment. The longer the patient is exposed to the HIV infection, the greater the damage to the gut, leading to susceptibility to opportunistic infections. Sharpstone and associates[23] determined that gastric emptying was delayed in patients with AIDS, absorptive capacity was reduced, and intestinal permeability was significantly increased in AIDS, presumably caused by prolonged HIV infection. Price and colleagues[24] evaluated a group of 22 patients infected with HIV on antiretroviral medication with chronic diarrhea and measured levels of fecal elastase. Eight of the 22 patients had fecal elastase levels less than 200 μg/g and found that those patients had symptoms of steatorrhea (fat in the feces) and weight loss. Fecal elastase is a digestive enzyme produced in the pancreas and low levels are used as a marker of pancreatic exocrine function.

Corroccio and colleagues[25] showed that, in patients infected with HIV with malabsorption, pancreatic enzyme supplementation was effective in reducing steatorrhea; however, this trial was conducted before the advent of HAART treatment protocols. Although the incidence of intestinal malabsorption has declined with HAART treatments, further research needs to be conducted to determine whether pancreatic enzyme treatments can improve intestinal functionality in patients infected with HIV.

Supplementation with prebiotics and probiotics has been proposed as a way to modify the environment in the large intestine and moderate the impact of inflammation and destruction of intestinal mucosa by the HIV virus. Results have been variable, with some patients having less drug-induced stomach pain and fewer lower gastrointestinal symptoms,[26] increased CD4 cell count,[27] or limited positive effects.[28] Research evaluating probiotic/prebiotic supplementation with macaques infected with simian immunodeficiency virus (SIV) showed that the supplementation resulted in increased number and functionality of acyl carrier proteins (ACPs) and functionality of CD4 T cells in the large intestine.[29] ACPs are involved in how cells signal and attach and can act as a tumor suppressor. These data further support the impact that an immunovirus (SIV) has on the gastric mucosa. Research using animal models provides an experimental environment in which protocol is closely followed and helps to provide an understanding of potential mechanisms of action.

Diarrhea is a common side effect and can be caused by medication side effects and diet intolerances. Dietary treatment of diarrhea includes consuming smaller, more frequent meals, and avoidance of gassy and spicy foods. Avoiding hot foods may also help slow gastric emptying time, whereas increased consumption of water and caffeine-free beverages is important to prevent dehydration. Foods with soluble fiber can help form the stool and should be increased as tolerated. These foods include oatmeal, applesauce, peas, avocados, and baked potato.

If cramping or bloating occur following ingestion of lactose-containing foods such as milk, then lactose-free milk and dairy products should be substituted. Lactase-reducing enzyme tablets are available over the counter and may also help with lactose intolerance. Caffeine and alcohol can also cause diarrhea and should be avoided to evaluate possible resolution of symptoms. If stools are foul smelling and float, fat malabsorption may be present. Changing to a low-fat diet or using prescribed pancre-lipase enzymes may help.[30] Risk of food-borne illness is greater during periods of infection, thus following established food safety guidelines during food preparation and handling can help prevent undesirable gastrointestinal symptoms that may contribute to weight loss.[30]

Keeping food safe from harmful bacteria that can further disrupt the gastrointestinal tract is crucial. Guidelines from the US Food and Drug Administration include cooking ground meats to an end-point temperature of 74°C (165°F) measured with a calibrated thermometer. Avoid consuming runny eggs; cook until firm. Use leftovers only once, heat to 74°C, and discard any remaining. Boil soups, gravies, and sauces before consuming.[30,31]

Hyperlipidemia

In a review article evaluating the lipid profile of patients infected with HIV,[32] the inves-tigators concluded that, "Patients with HIV/AIDS without ART (antiretroviral treatment) presented an increase of triglycerides and decreases of total cholesterol, low density lipoprotein (LDL-C), and high density lipoprotein (HDL-C) levels. Distinct ART regimens appear to promote different alterations in lipid metabolism. Protease inhibitors, partic-ularly indinavir and lopinavir, were commonly associated with hypercholesterolemia, high LDL-C, low HDL-C, and hypertriglyceridemia." Numerous other research articles have been published regarding lipid metabolism dysfunction[33,34] and various mecha-nisms of action have been proposed. Carpentier and colleagues[35] proposed the following mechanism: "the early development of hypertriglyceridemia frequently seen in HIV-infected patients treated with HAART occurs as the result of a combina-tion of a relative HAART-mediated increase in VLDL (very low density lipoprotein) secretion and an already impaired VLDL clearance."[35] In contrast, Pedersen and col-leagues[36] measured serum lipopolysaccharide (LPS) levels in patients infected with HIV versus noninfected controls as a biological marker of microbial translocation and found that "HIV-infected patients with suppressed viral replication had increased levels of microbial translocation as measured by LPS."[36] Higher LPS levels were asso-ciated with higher triglyceride levels, LDL-C levels, and insulin resistance, and these metabolic consequences tended to increase with time postinfection.

Regardless of the mechanism of action, changes in cholesterol and triglyceride metabolism seen in patients infected with HIV on HAART protocols need to be addressed. Pharmacologic treatment of high cholesterol levels in patients infected with HIV with statin drugs have been explored but interaction with various antiretroviral drug therapies may be impractical. Barrios and coworkers[37] evaluated the efficacy of a low-fat diet on cholesterol and triglyceride serum concentrations. A group of 230 pa-tients infected with HIV under HAART with dyslipidemia were included in a dietary intervention research study that lasted 6 months, and patients with good dietary compliance had reductions of cholesterol (10%) and triglyceride (23%) levels, whereas dietary noncompliant patients saw lesser reductions in cholesterol (2%) and triglyceride (9%) levels. Dietary supplementation with fish oil has been successful in reducing triglyceride levels in patients infected with HIV taking antiretroviral ther-apy,[38,39] with concomitant increases in both HDL-C and LDL-C levels. In a review[40] on the effect of omega-3 fatty acids (fish oil) on serum markers of cardiovascular dis-ease, the investigators noted that, in the 21 trials reviewed, levels of triglyceride decreased 27 mg/dL, HDL-C levels increased 1.6 mg/dL, and LDL-C levels increased 6 mg/dL. They concluded that the evidence supports a dose-dependent beneficial effect of fish oil on serum triglyceride levels, particularly among people with more increased levels. Several excellent reviews have been written on fish consumption and cardiovascular disease,[41] and triglycerides and cardiovascular disease.[42] A small pilot study evaluated the effect of extended-release niacin therapy (2000 mg/d maximum dosage) on patients infected with HIV with antiretroviral-associated dyslipidemia and noted significant reductions in serum triglyceride, total cholesterol, and non-HDL cholesterol levels. Even though the treatment regimen was well tolerated, 7 of 11 patients developed glucose intolerance (increased serum glucose level) after therapy and therefore this treatment protocol needs to have further research before widespread adoption.[43]

Lifestyle therapies should be included in the management of hyperlipidemia, with the main focus being selecting fat sources that do not exacerbate hypercholesterolemia or hypertriglyceridemia. Consumption of saturated fat should not exceed 7% of the total dietary caloric intake. Saturated fats are primarily found in animal products and selecting leaner cuts of meat and lower-fat or fat-free dairy products help to minimize their intake. Serum cholesterol levels should be less than 200 mg/dL and can be managed by selecting egg whites instead of whole eggs, more vegetables and fruits, and decreased consumption of animal products. Phytostanols and/or phytosterols in the diet have been shown to be effective nutritional supplements to aid in cholesterol reduction[44] as well as the addition of dietary fiber.[45] Total fat in the diet should be between 25% and 35% of the diet, with two-thirds of the fats coming from monounsaturated and polyunsaturated fats in a ratio of 2:1.[46]

Hyperglycemia

The incidence of diabetes mellitus in men on HAART infected with HIV treatment has been reported as being 4 times greater than that of men of similar age not infected with HIV,[47] whereas other epidemiologic studies have reported that, although HIV infection is not associated with the risk of diabetes, long-term treatment with antiretroviral therapies may increase the risk.[48,49] Yoon and colleagues[50] determined that a family history of diabetes, increased body mass index, and increased alanine transaminase levels were associated with the development of diabetes in individuals infected with HIV. Chehter and colleagues[51] found changes in the morphology in the pancreatic islet cells in patients with HIV receiving HAART compared with HIV treatment-naive patients. These changes could be contributing to the increased blood glucose levels seen in patients infected with HIV receiving HAART treatment. Other investigators have noted that pancreatic dysfunction may be related to the hyperlipidemia[52] seen in patients undergoing HAART, whereas Medapalli and colleagues[53] observed a correlation between patients with HIV with diabetes mellitus and chronic kidney disease.

Anderson and colleagues[45] in a meta-analysis report stated that, "for diabetic subjects moderate carbohydrate, high fiber diets compared to moderate carbohydrate, low fiber diets are associated with significantly lower values for postprandial plasma glucose, total and low-density lipoprotein cholesterol, high-density lipoprotein cholesterol and triglycerides." They recommend that the diet should provide 15 to 25 g of fiber per 1000 kcals of dietary intake. Patients prescribed steroids for HIV/AIDS therapy can develop hyperglycemia and steroid-induced diabetes.

Practical dietary recommendations to diminish hyperglycemia include reducing the level of simple carbohydrates (highly soluble carbohydrates) to less than 30% of the total carbohydrate intake and increasing the amount of unrefined low-glycemic-index (high-fiber) carbohydrate sources. Avoidance of concentrated sweets, such as candies, cookies, cakes, sugary drinks, and fruit juices, can assist with improving blood glucose control. High-fiber unrefined carbohydrate sources generate greater satiety than more highly refined versions and are also useful for individuals experiencing dyslipidemia.[45] Consumption of high levels of fructose or high-fructose corn syrup (HFCS) should be avoided. Recent studies with mice fed high levels of HFCS noted increased food consumption, obesity, and impaired insulin sensitivity,[54] whereas Basciano and colleagues[55] noted in their epidemiologic review that high dietary intake of fructose has become a major causative factor in the development of metabolic syndrome and dyslipidemia.

In addition, physical exercise is an important component in managing hyperglycemia. In a position paper published by the American Diabetes Association,[56] the following recommendation was promoted: "It must also be recognized that the benefit of physical activity in improving the metabolic abnormalities of type 2 diabetes is probably greatest when it is used early in its progression from insulin resistance to impaired glucose tolerance to overt hyperglycemia requiring treatment with oral glucose-lowering agents and finally to insulin."[56] There are many similarities between type 2 diabetic patients and individuals infected with HIV experiencing hyperglycemia. Management of hyperglycemia in individuals infected with HIV should follow a multipronged approach, including dietary management, pharmaceutical intervention, and increased physical activity when appropriate.

Oxidative Stress

Saeidnia and Abdollahi[57] stated that, "oxidative stress has been implicated in the progression of HIV to AIDS, since HIV usually replicates in a highly oxidized condition and $CD4^+$ T lymphocytes can be activated via a cascade of internal oxidative pathways involving inflammatory cytokines and enzymes."[57] Sharma[58] reports that the level of free radical species in individuals infected with HIV receiving "ART including HAART was reported to be higher than those who harbor HIV-1 without receiving any treatment or normal and healthy subjects." Managing the ratio of prooxidants to antioxidants is important in normalizing cellular homeostasis, and several reports have shown that antioxidant defenses (vitamin E, vitamin C, selenium, and coenzyme Q10) are compromised in HIV-positive patients compared with control populations.[59,60] Drain and colleagues[61] suggested that, "restoration of depleted micronutrients through supplementation may have several cellular and clinical benefits in HIV-positive patients receiving HAART."[61] Antioxidant and micronutrient supplementation have had variable results, with some investigators observing increased CD4 counts,[62] reduced oxidative stress,[63] or no response.[61] Forrester and Szlam[64] recommended that, "overall, dietary intake of micronutrients at RDA [recommended daily allowance] amounts remains a reasonable recommendation for persons with clinically stable disease. However, high-dose multiple micronutrient supplementation may benefit some persons with HIV/AIDS in the short term. Considerations include underlying nutritional status, immune status, the presence of coinfections, and whether the supplementation is intended for short-term rehabilitation or long-term maintenance."[64] Standard-dose oral vitamin and mineral supplements are recommended if diet is inadequate or lacks variety.[65] Recommendations for daily living are to increase the consumption of fresh fruits and vegetables in order to provide a varied complement of antioxidants and other bioactive compounds. Cocate and associates[66] noted that, "greater FV [fruit and vegetable] intake was independently associated with reduced [markers of inflammation] oxidized-LDL, 8-OHdG, and 8-iso-PGF2α in middle aged men."[66] General dietary guidelines include eating a variety of foods each day to obtain an array of vitamins and minerals.

Although most micronutrient and antioxidant requirements can be met with a varied diet of fruits and vegetables and a multivitamin supplement, vitamin D deficiency is becoming more prevalent in individuals infected with HIV.[67] Several studies[68,69] have noted a correlation between vitamin D levels and bone metabolism dysfunction (osteoporosis and osteopenia) in patients with HIV. It is not currently known whether the hypovitaminosis D is caused by ART/HAART therapy, malabsorption, disrupted conversion in the liver or kidney, or the lack of exposure to sunlight, but deficiency status needs to be addressed to avoid bone fragility. In addition, because vitamin D has recently been implicated in nonskeletal roles in the body,[70] including cardiovascular function, immune regulation, and anticancer properties, patients with HIV should be screened for vitamin D levels and supplemented if deficient.

SUMMARY

Nutritional counseling has been shown to improve dietary intake in individuals with HIV/AIDS.[71] Registered dietitians/nutritionists can individualize diet interventions to optimize effectiveness in treating metabolic consequences of the HIV infection or HAART. McDermott and colleagues[72] provided individualized nutrition counseling combined with commercial supplementation of 2 cans (8 fluid ounces, 240 total kcals, 15 grams of protein, 33 grams of carbohydrate and 6 grams of fat per can) per day and realized sustained improvements in dietary intake, body weight, and body composition. Subjects at baseline had numerous misconceptions, lacked sound nutrition knowledge, and were spending food dollars on unproven strategies. Emphasis was placed on food as medicine combined with behavioral strategies tailored to the individual's needs and clinical situation over a 12-week period. These interventions, along with guidance for having a food plan for sick days, resulted in overall improved dietary intake.

Nutrition management for individuals infected with HIV can be helpful in maintaining lean body weight, combating oxidative stress, reducing complications from hyperglycemia and hyperlipidemia, and managing gastrointestinal function but may need to be individualized to meet each individual's unique requirements. Consideration should be given to including the expertise of a registered dietitian/nutritionist as part of the health care team to promote wellness in the individuals infected with HIV.

REFERENCES

1. Samji H, Cescon A, Hogg RS, et al. Closing the gap: increases in life expectancy among treated HIV-positive individuals in the United States and Canada. PLoS One 2013;8(12):e81355.
2. The Antiretroviral Therapy Cohort Collaboration. Life expectancy of individuals on combination antiretroviral therapy in high-income countries: a collaborative analysis of 14 cohort studies. Lancet 2008;372:293–9.
3. Katona P, Katona-Apte J. The interaction between nutrition and infection. Clin Infect Dis 2008;46:1582–8.
4. Hommes MJ, Romijn JA, Godfried MH, et al. Increased resting energy expenditure in human immunodeficiency virus-infected men. Metabolism 1990;39: 1186–90.
5. Kosmiski LA, Kuritzkes DR, Sharp TA, et al. Total energy expenditure and carbohydrate oxidation are increased in the human immunodeficiency virus lipodystrophy syndrome. Metabolism 2003;52:620–5.
6. Mittelsteadt AL, Hilerman CO, Harris SR, et al. Effects of HIV and antiretroviral therapy on resting energy expenditure in adult HIV-infected women. A matched, prospective, cross-sectional study. J Acad Nutr Diet 2013;113:1037–43.

7. Hsu JW, Pencharz PB, Macallan D, et al. Macronutrients and HIV/AIDS: a review of current evidence. Consultation on nutrition and HIV/AIDS in Africa: evidence, lessons and recommendations for action. Durban (South Africa): World Health Organization; 2005. p. 10–3.

8. World Health Organization. Nutrient requirements for people living with HIV/AIDS, report of a technical consultation. Geneva, Switzerland: World Health Organization; 2003. p. 13–5.

9. Powanda MC, Beisel WR. Metabolic effects of infection on protein and energy status. J Nutr 2003;133:322S–7S.

10. Bernis K, Battegay M, Bassetti S, et al. Nutritional supplements combined with dietary counseling diminish whole body protein catabolism in HIV-infected patients. Eur J Clin Invest 2000;30(1):87–94.

11. Evans D, McNamara L, Maskew M, et al. Impact of nutritional supplementation on immune response, body mass index and bioelectrical impedance in HIV-positive patients starting antiretroviral therapy. Nutr J 2013;12:111.

12. Macallan DC, Noble C, Baldwin C, et al. Energy expenditure and wasting in human immunodeficiency virus infection. N Engl J Med 1995;333:83–8.

13. Mangili A, Murman DH, Sampini AM, et al. Nutrition and HIV infection: review of weight loss and wasting in the era of highly active antiretroviral therapy from the Nutrition for Healthy Living Cohort. Clin Infect Dis 2006;42:836–42.

14. Wilson IB, Roubenoff R, Knox TA, et al. Relation of lean body mass to health-related quality of life in persons with HIV. J Acquir Immune Defic Syndr 2000; 24:137–46.

15. Mwamburi DM, Gerrior J, Wilson IB, et al. Comparing megestrol acetate therapy with oxandrolone therapy for HIV-related weight loss: similar results in 2 months. Clin Infect Dis 2004;38:895–902.

16. Weiser SD, Young SL, Cohen CR, et al. Conceptual framework for understanding the bidirectional links between food insecurity and HIV/AIDS. Am J Clin Nutr 2011;94(6):1729S–39S.

17. Poles MA, Fuerst M, McGowan I, et al. HIV-related diarrhea is multifactorial and fat malabsorption is commonly present, independent of HAART. Am J Gastroenterol 2001;96:1831–7.

18. Knox TA, Spiegelman D, Skinner SC, et al. Diarrhea and abnormalities of gastrointestinal function in a cohort of men and women with HIV infection. Am J Gastroenterol 2000;95:3482–9.

19. Koch J, Garcia-Shelton YL, Neal EA, et al. Steatorrhea: a common manifestation in patients with HIV/AIDS. Nutrition 1996;12:507–10.

20. Garbonnel F, Beaugerie L, Abou Rached A, et al. Macronutrient intake and malabsorption in HIV infection: a comparison with other malabsorptive states. Gut 1997;41:805–10.

21. Wilcox CM, Waites KB, Smith PD. No relationship between gastric pH, small bowel bacterial colonization, and diarrhea in HIV-1 infected populations. Gut 1999;44:101–5.

22. Brenchley JM, Douek DC. HIV infection and the gastrointestinal immune system. Mucosal Immunol 2008;1(1):23–30.

23. Sharpstone D, Neild P, Crane R, et al. Small intestinal transit, absorption, and permeability in patients with AIDS with and without diarrhoea. Gut 1999;45:70–6.

24. Price DA, Schmid ML, Ong EL, et al. Pancreatic exocrine insufficiency in HIV-positive patients. HIV Med 2005;6:33–6.

25. Carroccio A, Guarino A, Zuin G, et al. Efficacy of oral pancreatic enzyme therapy for the treatment of fat malabsorption in HIV-infected patients. Aliment Pharmacol Ther 2001;15:1619–25.
26. Irvine SL, Hummelen R, Hekmat S. Probiotic yogurt consumption may improve gastrointestinal symptoms, productivity, and nutritional intake of people living with human immunodeficiency virus in Mwanza, Tanzania. Nutr Res 2011;31: 875–81.
27. Hummelen R, Changalucha J, Butamanya NL, et al. Effect of 25 weeks probiotic supplementation on immune function of HIV patients. Gut Microbes 2011;2(2): 80–5.
28. Schunter M, Chu H, Hayes TL, et al. Randomized pilot trial of a symbiotic dietary supplement in chronic HIV-1 infection. BMC Complement Altern Med 2012;12:84.
29. Klatt NR, Canary LA, Sun X, et al. Probiotic/prebiotic supplementation of antiretro-virals improves gastrointestinal immunity in SIV-infected macaques. J Clin Invest 2013;123(2):903–7.
30. Academy of Nutrition and Dietetics. Nutrition care manual. Available at: https://www.nutritioncaremanual.org. Accessed July 11, 2017.
31. US Department of Health and Human Services. Food and drug administration. Available at: https://www.foodsafety.gov. Accessed July 11, 2017.
32. Souza SJ, Luzia LA, Santos SS, et al. Lipid profile of HIV-infected patients in relation to antiretroviral therapy: a review. Rev Assoc Med Bras 2013;59(2):186–98.
33. Green ML. Evaluation and management of dyslipidemia in patients with HIV infection. J Gen Intern Med 2002;17(10):797–810.
34. Penzak SR, Chuck SK. Hyperlipidemia associated with HIV protease inhibitor use: pathophysiology, prevalence, risk factors and treatment. Scand J Infect Dis 2000;32(2):111–23.
35. Carpentier A, Patterson BW, Uffelman KD, et al. Mechanism of highly active anti-retroviral therapy-induced hyperlipidemia in HIV-infected individuals. Atherosclerosis 2005;178:165–72.
36. Pedersen KK, Pedersen M, Trøseid M, et al. Microbial translocation in HIV infection is associated with dyslipidemia, insulin resistance, and risk of myocardial infarction. J Acquir Immune Defic Syndr 2013;64(5):425–33.
37. Barrios A, Blanco F, García-Benayas T, et al. Effect of dietary intervention on high-ly active antiretroviral therapy-related dyslipidemia. AIDS 2002;16:2079–81.
38. Wohl DA, Tien HC, Busby M, et al. Randomized study of the safety and efficacy of fish oil (omega-3 fatty acid) supplementation with dietary and exercise counseling for the treatment of antiretroviral therapy-associated hypertriglyceridemia. Clin Infect Dis 2005;41:1498–504.
39. De Truchis P, Kirstetter M, Perier A, et al. Reduction in triglyceride level with N-3 polyunsaturated fatty acids in HIV-infected patients taking potent antiretroviral therapy. A randomized prospective study. J Acquir Immune Defic Syndr 2007; 44:278–85.
40. Balk EM, Lichtenstein AH, Chung M, et al. Effects of omega-3 fatty acids on serum markers of cardiovascular risk: a systematic review. Atherosclerosis 2006;189:19–30.
41. Kris-Etherton PM, Harris WS, Appel LJ. Fish consumption, fish oil, omega-3 fatty acids, and cardiovascular disease. Circulation 2002;106:2747–57.
42. Miller M, Stone NJ, Ballantyne C, et al. Triglycerides and cardiovascular disease. A scientific statement from the American Heart Association. Circulation 2011;123: 2292–333.

43. Gerber MT, Mondy KE, Yarasheski KE, et al. Niacin in HIV-infected individuals with hyperlipidemia receiving potent antiretroviral therapy. Clin Infect Dis 2004; 39:419–25.
44. Moreau RA, Whitaker BD, Hicks KB. Phytosterols, phytostanols, and their conjugates in foods: structural diversity, quantitative analysis, and health-promoting uses. Prog Lipid Res 2002;41:457–500.
45. Anderson JW, Randles KM, Kendall CW, et al. Carbohydrate and fiber recommendations for individuals with diabetes: a quantitative assessment and meta-analysis of the evidence. J Am Coll Nutr 2004;23:5–17.
46. Grundy SM. Nutrition in the management of disorders of serum lipids and lipoproteins. In: Shils ME, Shike M, Ross AC, et al, editors. Modern nutrition in health and disease. 10th edition. Baltimore (MD) and Philadelphia: Lippincott Williams and Wilkins; 2006. p. 1076–94.
47. Brown TT, Cole SR, Li X, et al. Antiretroviral therapy and the prevalence and incidence of diabetes mellitus in the Multicenter AIDS Cohort Study. Arch Intern Med 2005;165:1179–84.
48. Butt AA, McGinnis K, Rodriguez-Barradas MC, et al. HIV infection and the risk of diabetes mellitus. AIDS 2009;23:1227–34.
49. Tripathi A, Liese AD, Jerrell JM, et al. Incidence of diabetes mellitus in a population-based cohort of HIV-infected and non-HIV infected persons: the impact of clinical and therapeutic factors over time. Diabet Med 2014;31:1185–93.
50. Yoon C, Gulick RM, Hoover DR, et al. Case-control study of diabetes mellitus in HIV-infected patients. J Acquir Immune Defic Syndr 2004;37:1464–9.
51. Chehter EZ. AIDS and pancreas in the HAART era: a cross-sectional study. Int Arch Med 2014;6:28.
52. McGarry JD. Banting lecture 2001: dysregulation of fatty acid metabolism in the etiology of type 2 diabetes. Diabetes 2002;51:7–18.
53. Medapalli RK, Parikh CR, Gordon K, et al. Comorbid diabetes and the risk of progressive chronic kidney disease in HIV-infected adults: data from the Veterans Aging Cohort Study. J Acquir Immune Defic Syndr 2012;60:393–9.
54. Tetri LH, Basaranoglu M, Brunt EM, et al. Severe NAFLD with hepatic necroinflammatory changes in mice fed trans fats and a high-fructose corn syrup equivalent. Am J Physiol Gastrointest Liver Physiol 2008;295:G987–95.
55. Basciano H, Federico L, Adeli K. Fructose, insulin resistance, and metabolic dyslipidemia. Nutr Metab (Lond) 2005;2:5.
56. Zinman B, Ruderman N, Campaigne BN, et al, American Diabetes Association. Physical activity/exercise and diabetes mellitus. Diabetes Care 2003;26:S73–7.
57. Saeidnia S, Abdollahi M. Role of micronutrients and natural antioxidants in fighting against HIV; a quick mini-review. Res J Pharmacognosy 2014;1:49–55.
58. Sharma B. Oxidative stress in HIV patients receiving antiretroviral therapy. Curr HIV Res 2014;12:13–21.
59. Allard JP, Aghdassi E, Chau J, et al. Oxidative stress and plasma antioxidant micronutrients in humans with HIV infection. Am J Clin Nutr 1998;67:143–7.
60. Folkers K, Langsjoen P, Nara Y, et al. Biochemical deficiencies of coenzyme Q10 in HIV infection and exploratory treatment. Biochem Biophys Res Commun 1988; 153:888–96.
61. Drain PK, Kupta R, Mugusi F, et al. Micronutrients in HIV-positive persons receiving highly active antiretroviral therapy. Am J Clin Nutr 2007;85:333–45.
62. Kaiser JD, Campa AM, Ondercin JP, et al. Micronutrient supplementation increases CD4 count in HIV-infected individuals on highly active antiretroviral

therapy: a prospective, double-blinded, placebo-controlled trial. J Acquir Immune Defic Syndr 2006;42:523–8.

63. Jibril MM, Igbiks T, Atta AO, et al. Effects of micronutrients on oxidative stress in HIV positive patients taking highly active antiretroviral therapy (HAART) in a tertiary health care facility in Kano, northwest Nigeria. Bojapas 2016;9:99–107.

64. Forrester JE, Sztam KA. Micronutrients in HIV/AIDS: is there evidence to change the WHO 2003 recommendations? Am J Clin Nutr 2011;94(6):1683S–9S.

65. Isanaka S, Mugusi F, Hawkins C, et al. Effect of high-dose vs. standard-dose multivitamin supplementation at the initiation of HAART on HIV disease progression and mortality in Tanzania, a randomized trial. JAMA 2012;308:1535–44.

66. Cocate PG, Natali AJ, Oliveira Ad, et al. Fruit and vegetable intake and related nutrients are associated with oxidative stress markers in middle-aged men. Nutrition 2014;30:660–5.

67. Pinzone MR, DiRosa M, Malaguarnera M, et al. Vitamin D deficiency in HIV infection: an underestimated and untreated epidemic. Eur Rev Med Pharmacol Sci 2013;17:1218–32.

68. Arnsten JH, Freeman R, Howard AA, et al. Decreased bone mineral density and increased fracture risk for HIV infection. AIDS 2007;21:617–23.

69. García Aparicio AM, Muñoz Fernández S, González J, et al. Abnormalities in bone mineral metabolism in HIV-infected patients. Clin Rheumatol 2006;25:537–9.

70. Bikle D. Nonclassic actions of vitamin D. J Clin Endocrinol Metab 2009;94:26–34.

71. World Health Organization. Essential prevention and care interventions for adults and adolescents living with HIV in resource-limited settings. Geneva Switzerland: World Health Organization; 2008.

72. McDermott AY, Sheitz A, Must A, et al. Nutrition treatment for HIV wasting: a prescription for food as medicine. Nutr Clin Pract 2003;18:86–96.

The Role of Faith-Based Organizations in the Education, Support, and Services for Persons Living with Human Immunodeficiency Virus/Acquired Immunodeficiency Syndrome

Teresa M. Stephens, PhD, MSN, RN, CNE*

KEYWORDS

- HIV/AIDS • Resilience • Faith • Spiritual care • Social support

KEY POINTS

- HIV infection is a chronic health condition.
- Resilience is developed at any stage of life to help buffer the effects of stress and adversity.
- Faith and social support are key protective factors that can enhance an individual's personal resilience.
- Faith-based organizations are in a unique position to promote resilience in patients living with HIV/AIDS to buffer the effects of stress and adversity and to promote enhanced well-being.

INTRODUCTION

Individuals identified as resilient are known to possess certain protective factors that contribute to their ability to buffer the effects of stress and adversity. These protective factors are internal and external influences, and often include faith and spirituality. As the concept of resilience has evolved, it has been learned that it is something that is learned at any stage of life, leading to enhanced well-being and effective coping.[1–7]

Disclosure: The author does not have any financial interests to disclose.
College of Nursing, Medical University of South Carolina, 171 Ashley Avenue, Charleston, SC 29425, USA
* 487 Barr Road, Blountville, TN 37617.
E-mail address: Stephent@musc.edu

Nurs Clin N Am 53 (2018) 25–33
https://doi.org/10.1016/j.cnur.2017.10.003
0029-6465/18/© 2017 Elsevier Inc. All rights reserved.

Intentional efforts by faith-based organizations (FBO) to incorporate resilience-enhancing strategies for persons living with human immunodeficiency virus/AIDS (PLWHA) may effectively meet multiple needs of the individuals while simultaneously increasing their abilities to cope with future challenges, stressors, and transitions.

HIV-infected individuals now have a greater chance of living longer, because of advances in treatment, especially the use of antiretroviral treatments.[8] FBO are in a unique position to offer cost-effective community resources that lead to enhanced resilience and increased quality of life for the individual living with this diagnosis. FBO may provide important social and emotional connections that may lead to reduced anxiety and depression and improve cognitive and emotional function.[9] Additionally, faith and spirituality have been found to have a positive effect on the neurobiologic effects of stress. Decreased cortisol levels indicating a reduced allostatic load or reduced neuroendocrine consequence of stress have been shown in individuals who regularly attend church services, participate in prayer and Bible studies, and have higher levels of forgiveness toward perceived transgressions.[8-11] This article explores efforts by selected FBO to provide education, support, and services for PLWHA. Barriers, facilitators, and recommendations are discussed to encourage other FBO to begin addressing the needs of PLWHA as a natural progression of their ministries.

RESILIENCE

Resilient individuals have been described as those who not only survive, but also thrive following periods of stress and/or adversity.[1-3] As the concept has been further developed over the past few years and applied to multiple contexts, many researchers now agree that an individual may learn to develop or enhance his or her own resilience at any time in their lifetime.[1-7] Stephens[1] used the Norris' method of concept clarification to define nursing student resilience as "an individualized process of development that occurs through the use of personal protective factors to successfully navigate perceived stress and adversities. Cumulative successes lead to enhanced coping/adaptive abilities and well-being." Although resilience has most often been associated with periods of disaster or traumatic events, some researchers are beginning to explore the concept in healthy, well-adjusted individuals, particularly those experiencing life changes and/or transitions.[1,2,5,7,12] For these individuals, the concept of resilience is believed to help with everyday stressors and challenges, and the larger traumatic events most often explored in resilience literature.[12] The development of resilience assists individuals to better cope with everyday challenges, chronic illnesses, and life transitions and better prepare them for future stressors and possible adversity.[1,12]

Stephens' Model of Resilience (**Fig. 1**) includes five primary components: (1) perceived adversity, (2) protective factors, (3) interventions to increase protective factors, (4) cumulative successes, and (5) enhanced adaptive/coping abilities and well-being. Adversity and/or stress is perceived and processed by the individual based on previous experiences and current adaptive/coping abilities, which may be immature depending on the emotional development stage.[1] Protective factors are personal characteristics often found in individuals described as being resilient. Stephens' model proposes individuals are better equipped to manage stress and adversity as they learn to identify and enhance their personal protective factors. Cumulative successes lead to increased resilience and enhanced well-being.[1]

Interventions to increase an individual's protective factors can include formal educational programs and/or informal efforts, such as mentoring or personal

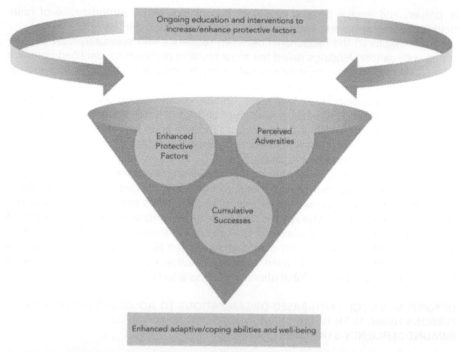

Fig. 1. The Stephens model of nursing student resilience. (*Adapted from* Stephens TM. Nursing student resilience: a concept clarification. Nurs Forum 2013;48(2):125–33.)

reflection. These interventions should be intentional and ongoing to reinforce the growth and development of personal resilience.[1–3,12] FBO can assist PLWHA in the development of resilience through strategic efforts aimed at the enhancement of specific protective factors identified through self-assessment and reflection. Even when efforts are not intentionally focused at increasing resilience, they often result in similar goals, as demonstrated by many FBO programs for individuals living with chronic illness.[13–16]

FAITH AS A PROTECTIVE FACTOR

Spirituality-faith is often cited in the literature as a helpful factor in coping with chronic disease/illness. Many individuals have noted the importance of their belief in God in helping them cope with adversity, maintain hope and optimism, and in managing their emotions.[13–16] Protective factors include individual (personal characteristics) and sociocultural (family and community) factors. Positive sociocultural influences contributing to protection include positive family support system (eg, connectedness with family members) and positive community support system (eg, resources, mentors, active participation, caring relationships with others).[1–4] Commonly identified protective factors include effective coping strategies, positive emotions, hope, faith, humor, self-esteem, confidence, optimism, perseverance/self-determination/drive, knowledge of health behaviors and risks, flexibility, self-efficacy, and sense of support/connectedness.[1–4] The role of faith and spirituality as they relate to health and well-being has been a topic of interest for many years. There is a plethora of research exploring the benefits of a personal belief in a higher power, the positive health effects of prayer, and similar protective factors associated with a strong sense of faith, including hope, optimism, and sense of purpose or meaning in life.[12–16]

Pentz[13] explored the relationship between resilience and spirituality-faith in older adults with cancer. Findings reveal the most resilient participants identified common themes related to their experiences with cancer, including (1) social support, (2) spirituality-faith (belief in God, hope, gratitude, helping others), (3) a positive attitude, and (4) positive coping.[13] The two major themes, social support and spirituality-faith, are applicable to the FBO seeking to engage and serve the PLWHA. Social support is often found through the natural activities of FBO and is an important buffer to stress during times of illness. Social support has also been found to assist individuals in finding meaning in their chronic illness.[13]

Despite the wealth of knowledge on the relationship between faith/spirituality and health and well-being, there is still a lack of services provided by FBO for PLWHA. There are many potential reasons for this, but much of the evidence points to a lack of knowledge about the disease process and the continued stigma toward PLWHA within the faith-based community.[17–26] Fortunately, there is much that is learned and replicated from FBO operating outside the United States. Many of these organizations are extensions of US-based churches or other FBO that have responded to the HIV/AIDS crisis through international missions efforts.[27–29]

OPPORTUNITIES FOR FAITH-BASED ORGANIZATIONS TO ADDRESS THE NEEDS OF PERSONS LIVING WITH HUMAN IMMUNODEFICIENCY/ACQUIRED IMMUNODEFICIENCY SYNDROME

According to the Centers for Disease Control and Prevention (CDC), the rates of HIV and AIDS are highest in the southern part of the United States, with African Americans having the highest percentage of HIV diagnoses. In 2015, the South accounted for 52% (9601) of the 18,303 new AIDS diagnoses in the United States. Additionally, southern states reported 53% (3570) of the 6721 deaths attributed directly to HIV or AIDS in 2014. Despite accounting for approximately 44% of all people living with an HIV diagnosis, southern states continue to lag behind other regions in some key HIV prevention and care indicators.[30,31] For this reason, much of the literature on the topic of FBO role in addressing the needs of PLWHA has come from African American FBO. Much is learned from these efforts to facilitate long-term impact on health through trusted and culturally competent HIV/AIDS interventions and support.

Because of the burden of geographic distribution of HIV/AIDS cases, the CDC has invested resources in the places and populations most affected by HIV, including the southern United States and African Americans.[30] These efforts include funding for state and local health departments, capacity-building organizations, and partnerships with community-based organizations representing some of the populations hardest hit by HIV/AIDS diagnoses.[17]

BARRIERS AND CHALLENGES

As HIV rates have continued to climb in the southeastern United States, particularly among African Americans, FBO have begun to recognize the need for action and participation in efforts toward prevention and support. Abara and coworkers[17] explored the challenges and lessons learned in implementing a faith-based community partnership to address HIV/AIDS in the southern United States. Southern African Americans were found to be particularly vulnerable to regional and racial disparities of HIV/AIDS because of complex challenges, such as stigma, normative attitudes and perceptions, and accessibility and availability of HIV testing resources.[17] According to the CDC, African American communities struggle with a disproportionate impact of HIV/AIDS.[31] For this reason, much of the literature on the topic of FBO role in HIV/AIDS services has come from the African American faith community within and outside of the United States.[18,19,22,23,25–29] Much is learned from these efforts by other organizations wishing to serve this population within their own faith communities to facilitate long-term impact on health through trusted and culturally competent HIV/AIDS interventions and support.

FAITH-BASED ORGANIZATIONS' ROLE IN REDUCING FEAR AND STIGMA

Several FBO have developed promising strategies to engage a wide range of FBO to provide intervention and support services for PLWHA that are effective and congruent with the doctrine and teachings of the FBO.[25] Many leaders within churches and FBO have voiced their fear and/or apprehension in addressing the needs of PLWHA because of personal lack of knowledge, fear of upsetting members of the organization/congregation, and the difficulty in maintaining the theological principles while addressing some of the more sensitive moral (eg, sexual) issues often included in the care of PLWHA. Some FBO have found success in doing this by treating HIV/AIDS as a public health issue rather than a sexual and/or moral issue. Instead of an "all or nothing" approach, many are seeing the value in providing at least some of the basic education and/or services instead of ignoring it all together to avoid upsetting a few members of the congregation. Partnerships with public health agencies and health care professionals who are members of the FBO are helpful in providing referrals and counseling to address some of these other questions or issues.[18,19,22,26,27]

Spiritual elders, a type of peer mentoring, have been used within FBO to promote resilience in the elderly living with cancer. The concept of spiritual elders, as described by Pentz,[13] could offer many possibilities for the FBO seeking to serve the PLWHA. Spiritual elders are individuals who have themselves been diagnosed with cancer and demonstrated resilience through effective coping, positive emotional health, and successful sources of support while maintaining a strong faith and spiritual life.[13] The diagnosis of cancer provides a unique common identifier for the spiritual elders to demonstrate empathy and understanding of the specifics related to living with cancer, but also provides opportunities for mentoring and leadership to guide others in the path toward resilience. In this study, spiritually comfortable older adults with cancer were paired with others who were spirituality-minded, but struggling with their faith. These dyads provide mutual benefits, including an increased sense of purpose/meaning in life for the volunteer. Pentz[13] found that many of the participants in this study viewed the help received from the volunteer to be better than from a trained professional. Spiritual elders, a type of peer mentoring, could offer many possibilities for the FBO seeking to assist the PLWHA to increase resilience and overall quality of life. The same principles may be applied to the PLWHA. Those who have successfully navigated the challenges of the diagnosis and the intricacies of healthy living within that realm, all while maintaining their faith and spirituality, possess valuable qualities that may be useful to the FBO seeking to educate, support, and serve others with the diagnosis.[13]

Some organizations have found they already possess the capacity to provide many needed services for PLWHA, including prevention/education, testing, and support services.[25,26] Many of these FBO agree that it is of vital importance to train church leaders on HIV/AIDS topics to dispel any false beliefs and answer common questions. Some have found it helpful to partner with other churches and FBO to offer community workshops designed to educate leaders within the FBO or church. Others have hosted

HIV screening events as part of community outreach. Church-wide level approaches include using sermons and observational comments, including relevant content in brochures/newsletters/bulletins, and responsive readings designed to increase congregants' HIV awareness and to enhance unity.[26]

Storytelling is often used as a culturally appropriate way to share experiences. Role model story videos have been used to share the experiences of getting tested for HIV. These stories include testimonials from male and female role models to discuss the process of getting tested, from ambivalence to the benefits of doing, such as obtaining peace of mind (Berkley-Patton). These role model stories may also be shared in printed form for targeted groups to provide specific information on risk-reduction, testing, and/or support.[25,26]

FBO may also choose to use specific ministries within the organization as sources of inreach and outreach. Targeted groups may include youth, seniors, women, parents, singles, couples, food/clothing pantries, prison ministries, school programs, and athletic programs. Beyond video and printed materials, telephone tree messaging, text messaging, and social media have all been found to be effective methods of communication.[25,26]

RECOMMENDATIONS

Many African American churches, particularly those in the Southeastern United States, have made great progress in addressing the complexities of a faith-based approach to HIV/AIDS prevention, education, and treatment. Several of these churches have increasingly come to embrace functions outside of the typical focus of worship services and spiritual teachings. These functions include being a source of community life, acting as an agent of social change, and providing health promotion and disease prevention programs.[17] The success of these programs indicates a clear justification for FBO to embrace the call to address the needs of PWLHA. In describing the results of one such program, the researchers emphasize the importance of obtaining the support of organizational leadership to dispel any dissent among church members; promote buy-in from the congregation; and to project a unified front for the education, support, and services to PLWHA. Additionally, the creation of formal HIV care teams, composed of members from the general church congregation, existing health/welfare/support ministries, and the community, was found to be vital to the acceptance and success of the implementation process. These formal care teams were found to be in a good position to partner with other community-based HIV/AIDS resources and agencies to extend services beyond the church. Ongoing technical assistance and frequent workshops served to maintain open communication, sharing successes, challenges, and effective strategies. Of particular importance was the need to develop a format for delivering the HIV-related information in a faith-based setting to alleviate unease from members who were initially hesitant to embrace such initiatives. HIV/AIDS materials and messages were formatted in a targeted and culturally appropriate context without sacrificing the facts of the disease process. Church leadership intentionally clarified the objectives from the pulpit and by including relevant topics into other church functions, such as prayer breakfasts, youth group meetings, sermons, and newsletters. By modeling these behaviors, the pastors of the churches involved were able to promote acceptance and open dialogue and an elimination of fear, misinformation, and stigma within their individual congregations.[17]

Much research is needed to explore the development, implementation, and assessment of programs by FBO to address the needs of PLWHA. Specifically, there is a need to identify relevant theoretic models, cultural and contextual features that affect the program success, and studies to explore various methods for delivering the content and/or interventions. Many opportunities exist for seminary students to explore the possibilities of alliances between public health entities and FBO to serve PLWHA. The increased emphasis on interprofessional care and research is another avenue for research, education, and funding to promote collaborative work with health care professionals and those in the ministry.

SUMMARY

The Parable of the Good Samaritan is well-known with the Christian faith and often referenced when considering the behaviors related to kindness, compassion, and response to individuals in need. This parable, told by Jesus Christ in Luke 10: 25 to 37, describes the encounter between a severely injured traveling Jewish man and a Samaritan. Important lessons to be learned from this parable include the understanding of the extreme differences between the two main characters, the Samaritan and the Jewish traveler. The Jews and the Samaritans had a volatile relationship and usually avoided any personal contact with each other. In fact, the Samaritans were often considered to be oppressed by their Jewish neighbors. However, on this day, a Samaritan was the one who chose to respond to the injured Jewish man's needs, using his time, resources, and provisions for immediate and continued care.

This parable may be applied to the roles and responsibilities of FBO in addressing the needs of the PLWHA. The first consideration is the nature of the relationship between the injured man and the Samaritan. Contextually, these individuals represent groups who rarely interact and are often involved in disagreements. The act of crossing the road to deliver aide to the injured man violated all normal codes of behavior for the Samaritan. He simply acted on his personal values without regard to political correctness, group affiliation norms, or fear of ridicule or scorn by his community. Second, the Samaritan did not just leave the man after rendering aide. He demonstrated his commitment to the continued care even if he himself was unable to deliver it. By taking the man to someone who could deliver this care and personally assuming the responsibility for the cost of this care, he demonstrated a lesson in true compassion and a desire for promoting health and well-being without consideration of this individual's lifestyle, personal beliefs, nor his ability to repay.

Nursing has long been considered a practice that incorporates science with caring. How we respond to those in need is a true testament to our professional and spiritual callings. As we seek to practice holistically, providing care to the individual and the community, we must consider the opportunities for care that exist as members of FBO. Our knowledge, skills, and attitudes may be used to promote health, deliver education, provide care, and reduce stigma. Partnering with FBO makes sense and may prove to be one of the most beneficial efforts in addressing the complex and sensitive health needs of PLWHA.

REFERENCES

1. Stephens TM. Nursing student resilience: a concept clarification. Nurs Forum 2013;48(2):125–33.

2. Stephens TM. Increasing nursing student resilience [dissertation]. Knoxville (TN): University of Tennessee; 2012.

3. Ahern NR. Adolescent resilience: an evolutionary concept analysis. J Pediatr Nurs 2006;21(3):175–85.

4. Earvolino-Ramirez M. Resilience: a concept analysis. Nurs Forum 2007;42(2): 73–82.

5. Gillespie BM, Chaboyer W, Wallis M. Development of a theoretically derived model of resilience through concept analysis. Contemp Nurse 2007;25(1–2): 124–35.

6. Hodges HF, Keeley AC, Grier EC. Professional resilience, practice longevity, and Parse's theory for baccalaureate education. J Nurs Educ 2005;44(12):548–54.

7. Jackson D, Firtko A, Edenborough M. Personal resilience as a strategy for surviving and thriving in the face of workplace adversity: a literature review. J Adv Nurs 2007;60(1):1–9.

8. McCance KL, Huether SE. Pathophysiology: the biologic basics for disease in adults and children. 7th edition. St Louis (MO): Elsevier; 2014.

9. Brewer-Smyth K, Koenig HG. Could spirituality and religion promote stress resilience in survivors of childhood trauma? Issues Ment Health Nurs 2014;35(4): 251–6.

10. Danese A, McEwen BS. Adverse childhood experiences, allostasis, allostatic load, and age-related disease. Physiol Behav 2012;106(1):29–39.

11. Tartaro J, Luecken LJ, Gunn HE. Exploring heart and soul: effects of religiosity/ spirituality and gender on blood pressure and cortisol stress responses. J Health Psychol 2005;10:753.

12. Stephens T, Smith P, Cherry C. Promoting resilience in new perioperative nurses. AORN J 2017;105(3):276–84.

13. Pentz M. Resilience among older adults with cancer and the importance of social support and spirituality-faith. J Gerontol Soc Work 2005;44:3–4, 3–22.

14. Purcell H, Whisenhunt A, Cheng J, et al. "A remarkable experience of God, shaping us as a family": parents use of faith following child's rare disease diagnosis. J Health Care Chaplain 2015;21:25–38.

15. Santibanez S, Lynch J, Paye Y, et al. Engaging community and faith-based organizations in the Zika response, United States, 2016. Public Health Rep 2017; 132(4):436–42.

16. Whisenant D, Cortes C, Hill J. Is faith-based health promotion effective? Results from two programs. J Christ Nurs 2014;31(3):188–93.

17. Abara W, Coleman J, Fairchild A, et al. A faith-based community partnership to address HIV/AIDS in the southern United States: implementation, challenges, and lessons learned. J Relig Health 2015;54:122–33.

18. Stewart J, Rogers C, Bellinger D, et al. A contextualized approach to faith-based HIV risk reduction for African American women. West J Nurs Res 2016;38(7): 819–36.

19. Otey T, Miller W. A mid-south perspective: African American faith-based organizations, HIV, and stigma. J Assoc Nurses AIDS Care 2016;27(5):623–34.

20. Szaflarski M, Ritchey P, Jacobson C, et al. Faith-based HIV prevention and counseling programs: findings from the Cincinnati census of religious congregations. AIDS Behav 2013;17:1839–54.

21. Kang E, Delzell D, Chin J, et al. Influences of stigma and HIV transmission knowledge on member support for faith-placed HIV initiatives in Chinese immigrant Buddhist and Protestant religious institutions in New York City. AIDS Educ Prev 2013;25(5):445–56.

22. Moore D, Onsomu E, Timmons S, et al. Communicating HIV/AIDS through African American churches in North Carolina: implications and recommendations for HIV/ AIDS faith-based programs. J Relig Health 2012;51:865–78.

23. Cornelius J, Cornelius M, White A. Sexual communication needs of African American families in relation to faith-based HIV prevention. J Cult Divers 2013;20(3): 146–52.
24. Coleman J, Tate A, Gaddist B, et al. Social determinants of HIV-related stigma in faith-based organizations. Am J Public Health 2016;106(3):492–6.
25. Griffith D, Pichon L, Campbell B, et al. Your blessed health: a faith-based CBPR approach to addressing HIV/AIDS among African Americans. AIDS Educ Prev 2010;22(3):203–17.
26. Berkley-Patton J, Thompson C, Martinez D, et al. Examining church capacity to develop and disseminate a religiously appropriate HIV tool kit with African American churches. J Urban Health 2013;90(3):482–99.
27. Watt M, Maman S, Jacobson M, et al. Missed opportunities for religious organizations to support people living with HIV/AIDS: findings from Tanzania. AIDS Patient Care STDS 2009;23(5):389–94.
28. World Health Organization. Faith-based organizations play a major role in HIV/AIDS care and treatment in sub-Saharan Africa. 2007. Available at: http://www.who.int/mediacentre/news/notes/2007/np05/en/. Accessed June 14, 2017.
29. Ndirangu E, Evans C. Experiences of African immigrant women living with HIV in the U.K.: implications for health professionals. J Immigr Minor Health 2009;11: 108–14.
30. Centers for Disease Control. Engaging faith-based organizations. n.d. Available at: https://www.cdc.gov/globalhivtb/who-we-are/resources/keyareafactsheets/faith-based-organizations.pdf. Accessed June 14, 2017.
31. Centers for Disease Control. HIV in the United States by geographic distribution. n.d. Available at: https://www.cdc.gov/hiv/statistics/overview/geographicdistribution.html. Accessed June 14, 2017.

Mindful Living with Human Immunodeficiency Virus and AIDS

Behavioral Medicine for Patient Resilience and Improved Screening Practices

Kate Hendricks Thomas, PhD, MCHES[a],*, Justin T. McDaniel, PhD[b],
Aaron J. Diehr, PhD, CHES[c], Kyleanne Hunter, PhD[d]

KEYWORDS

• Mindfulness • Behavioral medicine • HIV screening • Holistic health

KEY POINTS

- The purpose of this study is to explore the specifics of complementary techniques used to treat adverse symptoms of human immunodeficiency virus (HIV) and AIDS that offer dual benefits in treatment and prevention, and to prevent disease spread by encouraging screening.
- Researchers downloaded data from the Centers for Disease Control and Prevention (CDC) 2015 Behavioral Risk Factor Surveillance System, state-level (n = 51) HIV screening rates for 2015 from the Henry J. Kaiser Family Foundation, state-level HIV diagnosis rates per 100,000 for 2015 (n = 51) from the CDC, and state-level control variables for the statistical analysis from the US Census Bureau and the US Department of Agriculture, including (1) poverty prevalence in 2015, (2) the percentage of state residents in 2015 without a high school diploma, and (3) the percentage of state residents in 2015 without a health insurance plan.
- Three regression models demonstrated that HIV diagnosis rates tended to be higher in states where mindful movement practices were prevalent because participation in such activities may influence the extent to which someone might closely monitor their health and, thus, be willing to be screened for HIV.
- Behavioral medicine practices can improve quality of life for participants living with chronic conditions such as HIV or AIDS.

Disclosure Statement: There are no connections or conflicts to disclose.
[a] Charleston Southern University, CSU College of Health Sciences, 9200 University Boulevard, Charleston, SC 29410, USA; [b] Southern Illinois University, 475 Clocktower Drive Mail Code #4632, Carbondale, IL 62901, USA; [c] HIV/AIDS Section, American Public Health Association, Public Health and Recreation Professions, Southern Illinois University, 475 Clocktower Drive Mail Code #4632, Carbondale, IL 62901, USA; [d] Josef Korbel School of International Studies, University of Denver, 2199 S University Boulevard, Denver, CO 80208, USA
* Corresponding author.
E-mail address: kthomas@csuniv.edu

Nurs Clin N Am 53 (2018) 35–46
https://doi.org/10.1016/j.cnur.2017.10.004
0029-6465/18/© 2017 Elsevier Inc. All rights reserved.

BACKGROUND

Improving longevity and quality of life with a diagnosis of human immunodeficiency virus (HIV) or AIDS can involve more than medical and pharmacologic interventions.[1] The purpose of this study is to explore the specifics of complementary techniques to treat adverse symptoms of HIV and AIDS that offer dual benefits treatment and prevention, as well as prevent disease spread by encouraging screening. Behavioral medicine therapy, often referred to as complementary integrative health practices or complementary and alternative medicine, are nontraditional modalities that are not mainstream pharmacologic or physical treatments (conventional western medicine) for the treatment of disease or suppression of symptoms.[2,3] Medical and public health professionals advocate the use of mindfulness-based practices in the prevention and treatment realms.[4] These treatment modalities vary measurably and include acupuncture, yoga, health coaching, mind-body therapies (meditation, guided imagery, and biofeedback), and tai chi or qi gong.[5] Common to all of these modalities is an emphasis on mental training to cultivate awareness and focused attention to movement synchronization with breath.[6]

Mindfulness interventions teach participants unique methods for improving their own ability to regulate their nervous system and calm the body's fear receptors.[7,8] Typically, such interventions involve still, seated meditation; physical movements of varying difficulty levels; and instructional seminars on individual peace, spirituality, and stress management.[9–11] A review of the literature on integrative health practices indicates the importance of mindful movement.[3] Such movement practices include repetitive motion that syncs physical exertion to breath and mental focus. Common modalities include Pilates, yoga, swimming, tai chi, drumming, martial arts, and more.[11] Much of the reason that mindfulness mitigates symptomology and improves health can be found in a study of the stress response.[12] The human body operates intelligently to produce appropriate reactions to life's stressors. A reactive response is necessary for self-preservation and survival. Cortisol and adrenaline fire the large skeletal muscles needed for evasion and shut down unnecessary functions such as the immune, reproductive, and digestive systems.[11] Until stress becomes chronic, the response does not cause ill effects or worsen any existing illnesses. However, when the body's response is constantly firing, inflammatory proteins become more present in the bloodstream.[13] A host of illnesses and inflammatory conditions have been related to this chemical imbalance caused by chronic stress, including cancer, depression, and chronic pain.[14] Mindfulness practices as part of a behavioral medicine routine have been successful for reducing the immediate and chronic effects of stress and enhancing overall health.[15]

Interventions using mindfulness have met with tremendous success and have been used to improve health outcomes in a variety of populations.[16] The research basis for specific somatic treatment protocols is broad. Mindfulness interventions have been highlighted in community setting studies as effective in reducing stress and anxiety,[17] and in individual case studies looking at mindfulness and mood recovery.[18,19] Chronic pain has also been successfully treated.[20] Importantly, for individuals living with HIV or AIDS, immune function has been shown to improve with behavioral medicine–style interventions.[21]

Although these less traditional methods are not normally designed to replace standard medical protocols, they enhance the effectiveness of both treatment protocols and prevention programs by giving patients the ability and agency to experiment and select healing tools that are often self-administered and used in less stigmatizing nonclinical environments.[22] The tie between mindfulness practices and patient resilience is strong,[23] and behavioral medicine's importance to individuals managing chronic diseases, such as HIV or AIDS, cannot be overstated.[24] These practices also encourage greater attention to physical health, in general, and to the role they could play in the general population to improve adherence to primary prevention activities, such as health screenings and basic prevention activities, is considerable.[25]

METHODS
Study Design and Data Collection

Secondary data for the present ecological study were downloaded from several sources. First, the authors downloaded data from the 2015 Behavioral Risk Factor Surveillance System, a nationwide telephone survey conducted by the Centers for Disease Control and Prevention (CDC).[26] Of singular interest from the 2015 survey was the question, to which 441,456 interviewees responded, "What type of physical activity or exercise did you spend the most time doing during the past month?" In total, 78 response options; that is, types of physical activity, were available to participants for the aforementioned question. The authors recoded the survey response options to discriminate between participants who regularly engaged in mindful movement practices and those who did not. Specifically, the mindful movement activities of Pilates, yoga, swimming in laps, tai chi, and karate or martial arts received a code of 1, whereas all other physical activities received a code of 0. After survey responses were recoded, data were aggregated to the state level (including Washington, District of Columbia [DC]) to create the following variable: the percent of state residents who regularly engaged in mindful movement practices in 2015 ($n = 51$). Second, we downloaded state-level ($n = 51$) HIV screening rates for 2015 from the Henry J. Kaiser Family Foundation.[27] Third, state-level HIV diagnosis rates per 100,000 for 2015 ($n = 51$) were downloaded from the CDC.[28] Fourth, we also downloaded several state-level control variables for the statistical analysis from the US Census Bureau and the US Department of Agriculture, such as (1) poverty prevalence in 2015,[29] (2) the percentage of state residents in 2015 without a high school diploma,[30] and (3) the percentage of state residents in 2015 without a health insurance plan.[31]

Data Analysis

To the extent that the present study used states in the United States as the unit of analysis, the creation of choropleth maps was possible. Using graduated symbols, 3 state-level choropleth maps were created in Q-GIS to represent 2015 data[32]: (1) the geographic distribution of regular participation in mindful movement practices, (2) the geographic distribution of HIV screening rates, and (3) the geographic distribution of HIV diagnosis rates per 100,000. Means, standard deviations, and percentages were also calculated for all study variables to generate a descriptive understanding of national results.

Meditation was tested using the procedures developed by Baron and Kenny.[33] Specifically, to determine mediation, they suggested that 3 regression models should be estimated. First, a model (Eq. 1) should be estimated to determine the influence of the independent variable (X) on the mediating variable (M). Second, a model (Eq. 2) should be estimated to determine the influence of X on the dependent variable (Y). Third, a model (Eq. 3) should be estimated to determine the influence of the X and the M on the Y. The following conditions must hold with regard to the 3 aforementioned models for perfect mediation to be evident: (1) there must be a statistically significant relationship between the X and the M in the first model, (2) there must be a statistically significant relationship between the X and the Y in the second model, and (3) the M (but not the X) must be a statistically significant predictor of the Y in the third model.

$$M_{ij} = \beta_{0j} + \beta_\alpha X_{ij} \tag{1}$$

$$Y_{ij} = \beta_{0j} + \beta_c X_{ij} \tag{2}$$

$$Y_{ij} = \beta_{0j} + \beta_{c'} X_{ij} + \beta_b M_{ij} \tag{3}$$

To test the mediating effect of state-level HIV screening rates (M) on the relationship between state-level prevalence of regular participation in mindful movement practices (X) and state-level HIV diagnosis rates per 100,000 in 2015 (Y), we estimated the previously described regression models using ordinary least squares.[34] State-level poverty prevalence, education levels, and health insurance coverage were entered as control variables in each regression model. Each regression model was bootstrapped with 1000 resamples to improve the precision of estimates.[35] The indirect effect, which specifies the amount of mediation in the model, was tested for statistical significance with MacKinnon, Lockwood, and Williams'[36] Monte Carlo Method for Assessing Mediation (MCMAM). In the MCMAM approach, "a sampling distribution of $\beta_\alpha \beta_b$ is formed by repeatedly generating β_α and β_b and computing their product ... [and] percentiles of this sampling distribution are identified to serve as limits for a $100(1 - \alpha)\%$ asymmetric confidence interval."[37(p83)]

RESULTS

Geographically based results for 2015 are shown in **Fig. 1**, **Fig. 2**, and **Fig. 3**. Regular participation in mindful movement practices was most prevalent in Washington, DC (3.60%), Hawaii (3.60%), New York (3.10%), Connecticut (3.10%), and Rhode Island (3.00%). Mississippi residents (0.70%) exhibited the least amount of participation in mindful movement practices. The national average, based on a calculation of an

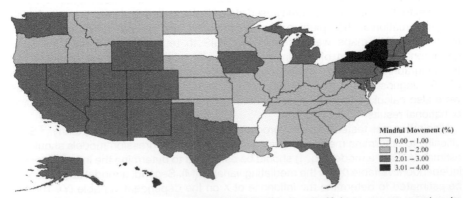

Fig. 1. Geographic distribution of regular participation in mindful movement practices in 2015.

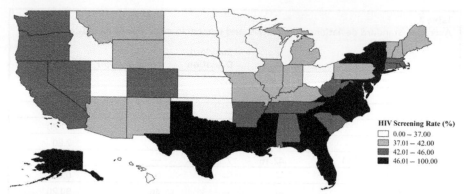

Fig. 2. Geographic distribution of HIV screening rates in 2015.

arithmetical mean of state percentages, for regular participation in mindful movement practices was 1.95% (**Table 1**).

In general, HIV screening rates were highest in the Gulf Coast and East Coast states, such as Washington, DC (75%), New York (55.50%), and Florida (51.10%). Utah exhibited the lowest state-wide HIV screening rate in 2015 (26.80%), followed closely by South Dakota (29.40%). Overall, the national HIV screening rate in 2015 was 42.16%. HIV diagnoses per 100,000 in 2015 were most frequent in Washington, DC (66.10), followed by Louisiana (29.20), and least frequent in New Hampshire (1.90). The average state-level HIV diagnosis rate per 100,000 in 2015 was 11.90 (see **Table 1**). Descriptive statistics for the 3 control variables, poverty prevalence, education level, and health insurance coverage, are shown in **Table 1**.

The results of the meditation analysis are shown in **Table 2**. Three regression models were estimated to determine whether state-level HIV screening rates mediated the relationship between regular participation in mindful movement practices at the state-level and state-level HIV diagnoses per 100,000 in 2015. In other words, testing was conducted to determine if HIV diagnosis rates tended to be higher in states where mindful movement practices were prevalent because participation in such activities may influence the extent to which someone might closely monitor their health and, thus, be willing to be screened for HIV. Three control variables were

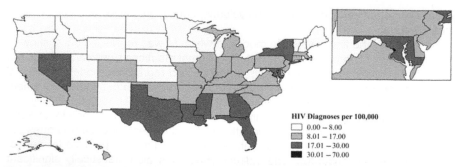

Fig. 3. Geographic distribution of HIV diagnoses per 100,000 in 2015.

Table 1
Averages, standard deviations, frequencies, and percentages of state-level indicators

	Mean	Standard Deviation	Frequency (n)	Percent (%)
Mindful Movement (%)	1.95	0.64	—	—
0.00–1.00	—	—	3	5.90
1.01–2.00	—	—	23	45.10
2.01–3.00	—	—	21	41.20
3.01–4.00	—	—	4	7.80
HIV Screening Rate (%)	42.16	7.99	—	—
0.00–25.00	—	—	0	0.00
25.01–50.00	—	—	46	90.20
50.01–75.00	—	—	3	5.90
75.01–100.00	—	—	1	2.00
HIV Diagnoses per 100,000	11.90	10.50	—	—
0.00–20.00	—	—	43	84.30
20.01–40.00	—	—	7	13.70
40.01–60.00	—	—	0	0.00
60.01–80.00	—	—	1	2.00
Poverty Prevalence (%)	13.72	3.54	—	—
0.00–6.00	—	—	0	0.00
6.01–12.00	—	—	21	41.20
12.01–18.00	—	—	23	45.10
18.01–24.00	—	—	7	13.70
No High School Education (%)	11.75	3.07	—	—
0.00–5.00	—	—	0	0.00
5.01–10.00	—	—	17	33.30
10.01–15.00	—	—	25	49.00
15.01–20.00	—	—	9	17.60
No Health Insurance (%)	8.72	3.17	—	—
0.00–5.00	—	—	6	11.80
5.01–10.00	—	—	26	51.00
10.01–15.00	—	—	18	35.30
15.01–20.00	—	—	1	2.00

entered into each equation: poverty prevalence, educational level, and health insurance coverage.

The results of the first regression model, in which M was regressed on X, showed that higher rates of participation in mindful movement practices significantly predicted higher HIV screening rates. The results of the second regression model, in which Y was regressed on X, showed that higher rates of participation in mindful movement practices significantly predicted higher HIV diagnosis rates per 100,000. Finally, the results of the third regression model, in which Y was regressed on X and M, showed that higher HIV screening rates significantly predicted higher HIV diagnosis rates per 100,000. To the extent that X was not statistically significant in the third model, perfect mediation was demonstrated. The indirect effect was also statistically significant based on the MCMAM approach: $\beta_\alpha \beta_b = 5.50$ (95% CI = 0.12–12.64) (**Fig. 4**).

Table 2
The mediating effect of human immunodeficiency virus screening rates on the relationship between mindful movement practices and diagnosis rates

	1[a]	2[a]	3[a]
	$X \rightarrow M$	$X \rightarrow Y$	$\{X,M\} \rightarrow Y$
—	β	β	β
Mindful Movement (X)	0.06 (0.03)[b]	7.29 (3.46)[b]	2.03 (1.58)
HIV Screening Rate (M)	—	—	91.61 (26.29)[b]
Intercept	0.15 (0.08)[b]	−27.54 (10.83)[b]	−41.61 (9.92)[b]
Control Variables	—	—	—
Poverty Prevalence	0.01 (0.01)	1.68 (1.30)	1.13 (0.70)
No High School Education	−0.01 (0.01)	0.10 (0.43)	−0.50 (0.86)
No Health Insurance	0.01 (0.01)	0.11 (1.02)	0.15 (0.41)
F (df)	6.05 (4, 46)	8.20 (4, 46)	26.96 (5, 45)
p	<0.01	<0.01	<0.01
R^2	0.35	0.42	0.74

[a] Bootstrapped with 1000 resamples.
[b] Statistical significance based on a 95% bias-corrected confidence interval.

DISCUSSION
Limitations

When considering the findings of this exploratory report, several limitations must be acknowledged. Secondary analysis of the 2015 Behavioral Risk Factor Surveillance System survey data, although providing a large, randomly-selected sample of respondents, limited the scope of questions that could be asked about mindfulness practices as a predictive variable. Data were self-reported, which could be problematic due to respondent recall or reluctance to truthfully answer sensitive, personal questions. However, the use of self-report in survey-based research in the field is both accepted and common.[38]

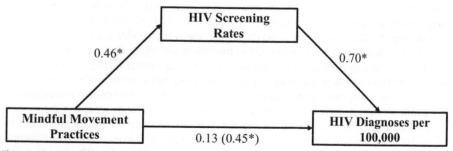

Fig. 4. Standardized regression coefficients for the mediating effect of state-level HIV screening rates on the relationship between state-level rates of participation in mindful movement practices and state-level HIV diagnosis rates per 100,000 in 2015. Asterisks indicate statistical significance based on a bootstrapped (with 1000 resamples) 95% bias-corrected confidence interval. The standardized regression coefficient between mindful movement practices and HIV diagnoses per 100,000, without controlling for HIV screening rates, is in parentheses.

SUMMARY

In 2015, nearly 40,000 people were diagnosed with HIV, and the rates of diagnosis varied by geographic region; specifically, the South had the highest rates at 16.8 (per 100,000 population), whereas the Midwest, at 7.6, had the lowest rates.[39] Collectively, the South also had the highest proportion of individuals living with HIV, accounting for 44% of all individuals in the United States living with HIV.[39] Lifetime risk for HIV diagnosis is also highest in the South, with the Washington, DC, presenting the highest risk; 1 in every 13 residents is expected to be diagnosed with HIV in his or her lifetime.[40] Among minority populations, the lifetime risk for HIV infection increases, with African American men having a lifetime risk of 1 in 20 and African American women having a 1 in 48 risk. Lifetime risk increases exponentially for gay and bisexual men who are racial or ethnic minorities. If current rates of diagnosis continue, 1 in every 2 black men and 1 out of every 4 Latino men who have sex with men will be diagnosed with HIV in their lifetimes.[40]

Although HIV screening rates tend to be higher than average in the South, specifically in the states clustered along the Gulf Coast,[27] southern states continue to display higher rates of HIV diagnoses. They also have disproportionately high rates of individuals diagnosed with AIDS, a diagnosis that has been linked with late testing and is seen more frequently among racial and ethnic minority populations, heterosexuals, and individuals with lower education levels.[41] Mortality among individuals with HIV is higher in the southern states as well. All but 2 states (Kentucky and Tennessee) exhibit higher mortality rates in individuals with HIV than the national average of 5.7 per 100,000 population.[27] Although the reasons for HIV-related disparities are multifactorial in nature, the experience of stigma, or the fear of experiencing it, can lead individuals to delay testing, avoid entering care, and not adhere to their treatment protocols.[42] Yet, studies have shown that reductions in perceived stigma can be achieved when individuals engage in mindfulness practices.[43–45] Incorporating these types of practices in geographic regions of the United States disproportionately affected by HIV could represent an approach to improving outcomes for individuals living in these areas.

In concordance with other smaller scale studies,[43–45] the results of the present study demonstrate correlation between improved screening behaviors and the practice of mindful movement protocols. As screening rates increased, diagnoses rates climbed. Gardner and colleagues[46] showed that for individuals to benefit most from HIV treatment, they needed to be screened, engaged in care, and adhere to their treatment plans. When individuals are engaged in treatment, their health outcomes improve dramatically. A CDC study that used data from the National HIV Surveillance System found that individuals actively engaged in treatment are highly likely to be prescribed antiretroviral therapy (92%), as well as achieve viral suppression (76%), meaning that the levels of HIV in a person's body are low enough to make transmission unlikely.[47,48]

Furthermore, early diagnosis and viral suppression allow HIV-positive individuals to have similar life expectancy as HIV-negative people. For example, a person diagnosed with HIV at age 20 and currently taking antiretroviral therapy would be expected to have a life expectancy similar to the general population,[49] whereas in the absence of HIV treatment, that same individual would only be expected to live 32 years.[47] Additionally, although undiagnosed HIV-positive individuals and individuals not in medical care were collectively linked to 91.5% of HIV transmissions in 2009 (30.2% and 61.3%, respectively); virally suppressed individuals were 94% less likely to transmit HIV.[50] As such, public health practitioners should continue to adopt novel approaches to increase screening levels and engage HIV-positive individuals in active treatment.

A strong evidence base exists for the recommendation of mindfulness practices for the general population because it improves rates of primary preventive practices and improves self-reported quality of life.[51] However, behavioral medicine can also improve quality of life for participants living with chronic conditions. In a systematic review of the literature, Carlson[52] found that mindfulness-based interventions were used to treat a variety of medical conditions, including HIV and AIDS, and that the findings suggested some level of benefit in most studies. In a randomized controlled study, HIV-positive individuals taking part in a mindfulness-based program showed improvements in stress, depression, and anxiety. Perhaps even more promising is that at follow-up they had significantly increased CD4 cell counts, a measure of immune system functioning that indicates improved health in individuals living with HIV.[53]

Evidence from studies of other vulnerable populations highlights that the community-building aspect of mindfulness activities encourages the participation in health-positive activities.[15,51] It is worth future study concerning the impact of community on individuals' decisions to engage in proactive health screening that enables them to receive early care The availability of mindfulness programming for people at risk for HIV should be a top concern for public health professionals working in the prevention and treatment spaces. Unfortunately, such programming is often offered by exclusive for-profit studios and is culturally inaccessible to socioeconomically disadvantaged parts of the country.[54,55] The exclusivity of such offerings creates massive barriers to benefit maximization.[56] Braveman[57] argued that, for health equity to be achieved, health must be framed in egalitarian terms; that is, it should be treated not as a luxury but as an inherent right. Improving availability, access, and cultural competency of behavioral health offerings could change the landscape of HIV and AIDS prevalence in many at-risk communities.[58]

REFERENCES

1. Rankin L. Mind over medicine: scientific proof you can heal yourself. Los Angeles (CA): Hay House, Inc; 2013.
2. Khoury B, Sharma M, Rush SE, et al. Mindfulness-based stress reduction for healthy individuals: a meta-analysis. J Psychosom Res 2015;78(6):519–28.
3. Thomas KH, Pence P, Huang J, et al. The physical dimension of recovery from invisible wounds of war. In: Seamone ER, Thomas KH, Xenakis S, editors. Invisible wounds of war. Cary (NC): Oxford University Press; in press.
4. Thomas KH, Albright D, editors. Bulletproofing the psyche: preventing mental health problems in our military and veterans. Santa Barbara, CA: ABC-CLIO/Praeger Publishing; in press.
5. Hendricks K, Turner L, Hunt S. Integrating yoga into stress reduction interventions: application of the health belief model. Ark J Health Promotion 2014;49:55–60.
6. Jha AP, Stanley EA, Baime MJ. What does mindfulness training strengthen? Working memory capacity as a functional marker of training success. In: Baer R, editor. Assessing mindfulness and acceptance processes in clients: illuminating the theory and practice of change. Oakland (CA): New Harbinger Publications; 2010. p. 207–21.
7. Meredith L, Sherborne C, Gaillot S, et al, editors. Promoting psychological resilience in the U.S. military. Washington, DC: RAND; 2011.
8. Nassif T, Norris D, Gomez M, et al. Examining the effectiveness of mindfulness meditation in combat veterans with traumatic brain injury. Washington, DC: American University; 2013.

9. Bearman D, Shafarman S. The Feldenkrais method in the treatment of chronic pain: a study of efficacy and cost effectiveness. Am J Pain Management 1999; 1999(9):22–7.

10. Ospina MB, Bond K, Karkhaneh M, et al. Meditation practices for health: state of the research. Evid Rep Technol Assess (Full Rep) 2007;(155):1–263.

11. Seaward B. Managing stress: principles and strategies for health and well-being. Sudbury (MA): Jones & Bartlett; 2004.

12. Hendricks Thomas K. Brave, strong, true: the modern warrior's battle for balance. Clarksville (TN): Innovo Publishing; 2015.

13. van der Kolk BA, McFarlane AC, editors. Traumatic stress: the effects of over-whelming experience on mind, body, and society. New York: Guilford Press; 2012.

14. Burchfield SR. The stress response: a new perspective. Psychosom Med 1979; 41(8):661–72.

15. Emerson D, Sharma R, Chaudhry S, et al. Trauma-sensitive yoga: Principles, practice, and research. Int J Yoga Therap 2009;19:123–8.

16. van der Kolk BA. The body keeps score: brain, mind, and body in the healing of trauma. New York: Penguin; 2014.

17. Thomas KH, Plummer Taylor S. Bulletproofing the psyche: mindfulness interventions in the training environment to improve resilience in the military and veteran communities. Adv Soc Work 2015;16(2):312–22.

18. Jouper J, Johansson M. Qigong and mindfulness-based mood recovery: exercise experiences from a single case. J Bodyw Mov Ther 2012;17(1):69–76.

19. Pence P, Katz L, Huffman C, et al. Delivering integrative restoration-yoga nidra meditation (iRest®) to women with sexual trauma at a veteran's medical center: a pilot study. Int J Yoga Therap 2014;24(1):53–62.

20. Smeeding SJ, Bradshaw DH, Kumpfer K, et al. Outcome evaluation of the Veterans Affairs Salt Lake City Integrative Health Clinic for chronic pain and stress-related depression, anxiety, and post-traumatic stress disorder. J Altern Complement Med 2010;16(8):823–35.

21. Wang M, An L. Effects of 12 weeks' tai chi chuan practice on the immune function of female college students who lack physical exercise. Biol Sport 2011;28(1): 45–9.

22. Barrett B. Alternative, complementary, and conventional medicine: is integration upon us? J Altern Complement Med 2003;9(3):417–27.

23. Thomas KH, Turner LW, Kaufman E, et al. Predictors of depression diagnoses and symptoms in veterans: results from a national survey. Mil Beh Health 2015; 3(4):255–65.

24. Richardson G. The metatheory of resilience and resiliency. J Clin Psychol 2002; 58(3):307–21.

25. Becker I. Uses of yoga in psychiatry and medicine. In: Muskin PR, editor. Complementary and alternative medicine and psychiatry. Washington, DC: American Psychiatric Press, Inc; 2008. p. 107–46.

26. Centers for Disease Control and Prevention. 2015 BRFSS survey data and documentation. Available at: https://www.cdc.gov/brfss/annual_data/annual_2015.html. Accessed April 19, 2017.

27. Henry J. Kaiser Family Foundation. State health facts. Available at: http://kff.org/state-category/hivaids/. Accessed April 19, 2017.

28. Center for Disease Control and Prevention. HIV in the United States by geographic distribution. Available at: https://www.cdc.gov/hiv/statistics/overview/geographicdistribution.html. Accessed April 19, 2017.

29. United States Census Bureau. Income and poverty in the United States: 2015. Available at: https://www.census.gov/data/tables/2016/demo/income-poverty/p60-256.html. Accessed April 19, 2017.

30. United States Department of Agriculture. County level data sets. Available at: https://data.ers.usda.gov/reports.aspx?ID=18243. Accessed April 19, 2017.

31. United States Census Bureau. Health insurance in the United States: 2015 tables. Available at: https://www.census.gov/data/tables/2016/demo/health-insurance/p60-257.html. Accessed April 19, 2017.

32. QGIS Development Team. QGIS geographic information system version 2.14. Available at: http://qgis.com. Accessed August 20, 2016.

33. Baron R, Kenny DA. The moderator-mediator variable distinction in social psychological research: conceptual, strategic, and statistical considerations. J Pers Soc Pyschol 1986;51:1173–82.

34. Long RG. The crux of the method: assumptions in ordinary least squares and logistic regression. Psychol Rep 2008;103(2):431–4.

35. Freedman DA. Bootstrapping regression models. Ann Stat 1981;6:1218–28.

36. MacKinnon DP, Lockwood CM, Williams J. Confidence limits for the indirect effect: distribution of the product and resampling methods. Multivariate Behav Res 2004;39:99–128.

37. Preacher KJ, Selig JP. Advantages of Monte Carlo confidence intervals for indirect effects. Comm Methods Meas 2012;6:77–98.

38. Alvarez J, Canduela J, Raeside R. Knowledge creation and the use of secondary data. J Clin Nurs 2012;21(19):2699–710.

39. Centers for Disease Control and Prevention. HIV surveillance report, 2015. Atlanta (GA): US Department of Health and Human Services; 2016. Available at. https://www.cdc.gov/hiv/pdf/library/reports/surveillance/cdc-hiv-surveillance-report-2015-vol-27.pdf.

40. Centers for Disease Control and Prevention. Lifetime risk of HIV diagnosis. Available at: https://www.cdc.gov/nchhstp/newsroom/2016/croi-press-release-risk.html. Accessed June 16, 2017.

41. Centers for Disease Control and Prevention. Late versus early testing of HIV—16 sites, United States, 2000-2003. MMWR Morb Mortal Wkly Rep 2003;52(25):581–6.

42. Chesney MA, Smith AW. Critical delays in HIV testing and care. Am Behav Sci 1999;42(7):1162–74.

43. Brion JM, Menke EM. Perspectives regarding adherence to prescribed treatment in highly adherent HIV-infected gay men. J Assoc Nurses AIDS Care 2008;19(3):181–91.

44. Brion JM, Leary MR, Drabkin AS. Self-compassion and reactions to serious illness: the case of HIV. J Health Psychol 2014;19(2):218–29.

45. Yang X, Mak WWS. The differential moderating roles of self-compassion and mindfulness in self-stigma and well-being among people living with mental illness or HIV. Mindfulness N Y 2017;8(3):595–602.

46. Gardner EM, McLees MP, Steiner JF, et al. The spectrum of engagement in HIV care and its relevance to test-and-treat strategies for prevention of HIV infection. Clin Infect Dis 2011;52(6):793–800.

47. Centers for Disease Control and Prevention. HIV care saves lives. Available at: https://www.cdc.gov/vitalsigns/hiv-aids-medical-care/index.html. Accessed June 16, 2017.

48. Bradley H, Hall HI, Wolitski RJ, et al. Vital signs: HIV diagnosis, care, and treatment among persons living with HIV—United States, 2011. MMWR Morb Mortal Wkly Rep 2014;63(47):1113–7.
49. Samji H, Cescon A, Hogg RS, et al. Closing the gap: Increases in life expectancy among treated HIV-positive individuals in the United States and Canada. PLoS One 2013;8(12):e81355.
50. Skarbinski J, Rosenberg E, Paz-Bailey G. Human immunodeficiency virus transmission at each step of the care continuum in the United States. JAMA Intern Med 2015;175(4):588–96.
51. Thomas KH, Plummer Taylor S, Hamner K, et al. Multi-site programming offered to promote resilience in military veterans: a process evaluation of the just roll with it bootcamps. Calif J Health Promot 2015;13(2):15–24.
52. Carlson LE. Mindfulness-based interventions for physical conditions: a narrative review evaluating levels of evidence. ISRN Psychiatry 2012. https://doi.org/10.5402/2012/651583.
53. Gonzalez-Garcia M, Ferrer MJ, Borras X, et al. Effectiveness of mindfulness-based cognitive therapy on the quality of life, emotional status, and CD4 cell counts of patients aging with HIV infection. AIDS Behav 2014;18(4):676–85.
54. Horton C. 21st century yoga: culture, politics, and practice. Chicago: Kleio Books; 2012.
55. Mostafa-Kamel S. Taking yoga off our mat: approaching Montreal's yoga culture with a critical lens. (Doctoral dissertation). Montreal (QC): McGill University; 2014.
56. Brown JLC, Eubanks C, Keating A. Yoga, quality of life, anxiety, and trauma in low-income adults with mental illness: a mixed-methods study. Social Work Ment Health 2016;15(3):1–23.
57. Braveman P. Health disparities and health equity: concepts and measurement. Annu Rev Public Health 2006;27:167–94.
58. Davis-Berman J. Contributing cause of death: poverty. J Soc Work End Life Palliat Care 2013;9(4):244–6.

Promoting Cardiovascular Health in Patients Living with Human Immunodeficiency Virus/Acquired Immunodeficiency Syndrome

CrossMark

Robin Harris, PhD, ANP-BC, ACNS-BC

KEYWORDS

- HIV/AIDS • Cardiovascular disease • Cardiomyopathy • Coronary disease

KEY POINTS

- Human immunodeficiency virus infection is a chronic health condition.
- Cardiovascular disease has increased in patients living with human immunodeficiency virus/acquired immunodeficiency syndrome (PLWHA) because of increased life expectancy.
- Early detection and treatment of cardiovascular disease is essential for health promotion in PLWHA.

INTRODUCTION

Approximately 37 million people around the world are living with human immunodeficiency virus (HIV).[1] HIV infection alters normal immune system function and can progress to advanced-stage acquired immunodeficiency syndrome (AIDS). Since the beginning of the HIV/AIDS epidemic in the 1980s, more than 35 million HIV/AIDS-related deaths have been reported.[2] Worldwide, close to 1.1 million people died of HIV/AIDS-related causes in 2015.[3] Sub-Saharan Africa has the highest number of patients with AIDS and the highest number of new cases of HIV infection diagnosed each year, accounting for 65% of all new cases of HIV diagnosis annually.[2] In the United States, new cases of HIV infection decreased 18% from 2008 to 2014.[3] It is estimated that there are 1.1 million adults and children in the United States living with HIV infection. A reported 15% of individuals with HIV infection in the United States are unaware of their HIV status and are undiagnosed.[3]

Disclosure: The author has no financial interests to disclose.
College of Nursing, University of Tennessee, 1200 Volunteer Boulevard, Knoxville, TN 37996, USA
E-mail address: rharri24@utk.edu

Nurs Clin N Am 53 (2018) 47–56
https://doi.org/10.1016/j.cnur.2017.10.005
nursing.theclinics.com
0029-6465/18/© 2017 Elsevier Inc. All rights reserved.

Despite research and advances in treatment of individuals with HIV infection, there remains no cure for this disease. Use of antiretroviral treatments (ART) has decreased HIV-related morbidity and mortality because of effects on viral replication and progression of the disease to AIDS.[4] The World Health Organization (WHO) reports that 18.2 million people worldwide were receiving ART by mid-2016.[2] Access to ART could prevent an estimated 21 million deaths and 28 million new cases of HIV/AIDS by 2030.[2] Current evidence-based guidelines recommend use of ART for all individuals infected with HIV regardless of age or CD4+ cell count.[1,2]

As HIV-related morbidity and mortality have decreased with the use of ART, the number of people living with HIV/AIDS (PLWHA) has increased.[1] With increased life expectancy, the effects of HIV infection on major body systems and resulting heart, lung, and blood diseases have become more apparent.[5,6] Cardiovascular disease conditions, including dyslipidemia, coronary artery disease, peripheral vascular disease, cardiomyopathy, cardiac arrhythmias, myocardial disease, pericardial disease, and valvular disease, have increased in PLWHA as a result of the direct effects of the HIV virus on cardiovascular tissue and the effects of ART regimens.[1,7,8] An overview of the effects of the HIV virus and ART on the cardiovascular system is presented in this article.

HISTORY

The earliest cases of HIV/AIDS were first identified in the early 1980s. All early cases were similar in presentation with pulmonary infection and profound immune deficiency. The extreme immune deficiency was determined to be from a viral infection identified as a retrovirus and named HIV. Unlike other viruses, a retrovirus has its genetic transcription on 2 copies of a single RNA strand rather than on double-stranded DNA.[4] The HIV retrovirus gains access to the immune system by invading CD4+ T-helper cells. Through a multistep process, the enzyme reverse transcriptase converts single-strand viral RNA to double-strand DNA, which is then integrated via the enzyme integrase into the genetic DNA molecule of the host cell. New viral cells can form in the host cell and cause lysis of the host cell and release of the newly formed viral particles if the host cell is activated. The host cell may also remain dormant and the viral particles latent for an extended period of time. The enzyme protease is required for final protein synthesis and maturation of the newly formed viral cells within the host cell.[9] As newly formed HIV viral cells are released into the blood stream, invasion of CD4+ T-helper cells by the HIV virus continues and results in altered immune system response. The immune system becomes overwhelmed and unable to protect itself from the HIV virus and invasion from other opportunistic micoorganisms.[4] The time from HIV infection to development of clinical symptoms is variable and is reported to be as long as 10 years in some individuals.[10]

The first antiretroviral drug, zidovudine, was introduced in 1987.[11] Initial treatment response to antiretroviral medication in patients infected with HIV was encouraging. However, viral resistance developed and zidovudine as a single agent became less effective against HIV infection. A new antiretroviral drug class, protease inhibitors (PIs), was first introduced in the 1990s.[11] Additional new drugs classes introduced during this time targeted different steps in the HIV infection process. The new antiretroviral drugs, known as highly active ART, were more effective in controlling HIV viral replication and progression.[9]

At present, there are 6 classes of antiretroviral drugs available that target different steps in the HIV viral infection and replication process. Reverse transcriptase inhibitors block the effects of the enzyme reverse transcriptase necessary for transcription of viral RNA into host cell DNA. The reverse transcriptase inhibitor class of antiretroviral drugs can be further divided into 2 groups: (1) nucleoside/nucleotide reverse transcriptase inhibitors (NRTIs), and (2) nonnucleoside reverse transcriptase inhibitors (NNRTIs).[9] PIs are effective by blocking the enzyme protease, required for final viral cell maturation. Integrase inhibitors block the enzyme integrase, which is required for the integration of HIV virus DNA into the host cell DNA. NRTIs, NNRTIs, and PIs are effective because they interrupt the processes involved in HIV virus replication.[9] In addition to agents that block HIV viral replication, pharmacologic agents are available that target a different step of HIV infection and prevent entry of the HIV virus into the host cell. Categories of antiretroviral medications that block the entry of the HIV virus into the host cell include HIV fusion inhibitors and chemokine receptor 5 antagonists.[9] Use of multiple agents that attack viral invasion and viral replication at different stages has improved response to treatment. Current guidelines recommend combined antiretroviral therapy (cART), defined as the use of at least 3 antiretroviral agents, consisting of 2 drugs from the NRTI class and 1 drug from another drug class.[12]

Before the use of cART, opportunistic infections and malignant cancerous processes were the most common causes of death in individuals with HIV infection that progressed to AIDS.[1] Life expectancy has increased with the use of cART, and HIV is now recognized as a chronic health condition.[1,12] PLWHA may live many years without progression of the viral infection to the advanced immune deficiency associated with AIDS. Increased life expectancy in HIV infection is associated with increased prevalence of cardiovascular disease in this patient population. The increase in cardiovascular disease is caused by direct effects of HIV viral infection on the cardiovascular system, use of cART treatment regimens and side effects, and presence of multiple cardiovascular risk factors in patients who are living longer.[1] Patients with HIV infection are at increased risk of cardiovascular disease and related complications regardless of the presence of HIV-related clinical symptoms. Use of multiple-drug treatment regimens has been effective to decrease HIV/AIDS-related hospitalizations. However, hospitalizations for non–HIV/AIDS-related chronic conditions, such as cardiovascular and respiratory illnesses, have increased.[13] Chronic cardiovascular disease conditions associated with non–HIV/AIDS-related hospitalizations include heart failure, hypertension, coronary heart disease, and stroke. African American patients living with HIV have a higher incidence of hospitalizations for heart failure and hypertension. White patients living with HIV have a higher incidence of hospitalizations for heart failure and stroke.[13]

CARDIOVASCULAR PATHOPHYSIOLOGY

HIV-positive patients are at increased risk of ischemic and nonischemic cardiovascular disease[14] (**Box 1**). Ischemic cardiovascular disease in HIV-positive patients includes coronary artery disease and peripheral vascular disease.[15] Nonischemic cardiovascular diseases include cardiomyopathy, pericardial disease, endocardial disease, valvular disease, pulmonary hypertension, and vasculopathy of the great and peripheral arteries.[7,8] Vascular diseases in PLWHA are primarily in individuals who are immunocompromised in advanced-stage disease and include infectious arteritis, inflammatory vasculitis, microvascular thrombosis, pulmonary hypertension, and venous thrombosis.[15] The underlying pathophysiologic processes of ischemic and nonischemic cardiovascular diseases are discussed here.

Box 1
Cardiovascular disorders and disease in human immunodeficiency virus/acquired immunodeficiency syndrome

- Ischemic disorders
  - Coronary artery disease
  - Peripheral arterial disease
- Nonischemic disorders
  - Cardiomyopathy
  - Myocardial disease
  - Endocardial disease
  - Pericardial disease
  - Vascular disease
- Increased risk:
  - Myocardial infarction
  - Acute coronary syndrome
  - Silent ischemia
  - Stroke
  - Limb ischemia
  - Heart failure
  - Pericarditis
  - Pericardial effusion
  - Valvular diseases
  - Cardiac arrhythmias
  - Pulmonary hypertension
  - Disease of great vessels
  - Peripheral vascular disease

Ischemic Cardiovascular Disease

The processes of inflammation and immune system dysfunction in HIV infection contribute to the development of cardiovascular disease.[1] Chronic systemic and vascular inflammation and immune activation are stimulated by activated T cells and monocytes. Inflammation at the vessel wall and activation of the immune system T cells, monocytes, and cytokines lead to formation of atherosclerotic plaques.[16] Overall risk for development of cardiovascular disease is 1.5 to 2.0 times higher in HIV-positive individuals compared with the general population.[1] Risk of myocardial infarction (MI) is higher in HIV-positive individuals with low CD4+ cell counts.[1]

Multiple studies have shown that coronary artery disease is associated with increased risk of MI in individuals infected with HIV.[12] In HIV infection, coronary arterial disease occurs as a result of inflammation at the vessel wall, endothelial dysfunction, and disorders in blood coagulation.[1] Development of atherosclerotic plaques in the coronary arteries can lead to narrowing of the arterial lumen, affecting blood flow through the lumen.[17] Atherosclerotic plaques in individuals infected with HIV are typically noncalcified plaques.[1] These noncalcified plaques are vulnerable plaques that are more likely to spontaneously rupture with subsequent development of thrombus resulting in a cardiac event.[18] With plaque rupture, myocardial ischemia and infarction can occur if blood flow is not returned to the tissue. HIV infection is associated with increased risk of MI.[1] Noncalcified plaques are more common in patients infected with HIV with lower CD4+ cell counts.[19] Incidence of MI has been documented at 50 years of age in HIV infection compared with ages greater than 60 years of age in patients not infected with HIV.[14]

The immune system plays an important role in inflammatory processes. Inflammation can be monitored by the presence of inflammatory markers, such as C-reactive protein (CRP). Other inflammatory markers that can be measured include interleukin-6 and tumor necrosis factor. Increased inflammatory marker levels are associated with increased viral load and increased cardiovascular risk.[1,16]

Use of biomarkers for inflammation has been shown to be useful in PLWHA to determine the risk of cardiovascular disease.[20] HIV-positive patients with increased CRP levels and inflammation are at increased risk of MI.[1] Inflammation affects normal endothelial function, causing disruption in the smooth endothelial vessel lining. Alteration in normal endothelial function is associated with atherosclerosis and cardiac events.[21] Inflammatory processes in combination with endothelial dysfunction result in progression of atherosclerosis in the coronary and peripheral arteries and increased risk of ischemic complications.[22] Risk of MI is further increased by the coagulation disorders that are common in individuals infected with HIV from chronic platelet activation and increased levels of blood clotting factors. Protein S deficiency and hyperhomocysteinemia have been documented in HIV-positive patients. HIV infection has been associated with higher levels of D dimer, factor VII, von Willebrand, and tissue factors seen in blood coagulation disorders.[12]

In addition to the inflammation, immune system responses, and coagulation disorders in HIV-positive patients, presence of cardiovascular risk factors, including tobacco use, hypertension, obesity, insulin resistance, metabolic syndrome, and dyslipidemia, further increases the risk of cardiovascular events in PLWHA.[1,5,8] Risk of cardiovascular disease is further increased by antiretroviral agents used in treatment of HIV infection. Dyslipidemia and increased risk for MI have been documented in HIV-positive patients treated with PIs.[12] PIs are associated with increased cholesterol and triglyceride levels. Other adverse effects of PIs include hyperglycemia/diabetes, lipodystrophy or fat redistribution, reduced bone mineral density, increased bleeding tendency in hemophilia, and increased serum transaminase level.[9] In addition to PIs, some NRTIs and NNRTIs can cause dyslipidemia and insulin resistance.[12] Side effects of ART include increased incidence of metabolic syndrome and MI risk.[23] In the absence of ART, the HIV virus has independently been shown to increase triglyceride levels and decrease high-density lipoprotein cholesterol (HDL-C) levels. The Strategies for Management of Antiretroviral Therapy (SMART) trial showed a higher rate of cardiovascular events in patients infected with HIV who had discontinued ART compared with patients infected with HIV who continued treatment.[14] Antiretroviral medications have been shown to alter HIV disease progression. PIs are associated with higher incidence of cardiovascular disease development caused by lipodystrophy, hyperlipidemia, and hyperglycemia side effects from these medications.[9]

Nonischemic Cardiovascular Disease

Cardiomyopathy in patients infected with HIV can occur from nonischemic causes, including the HIV virus, opportunistic viral infections, cancer, and medication side effects. Ischemic heart disease can also lead to cardiomyopathy in patients infected with HIV.[8] HIV infection results in chronic inflammation and alterations in the immune system response. Cardiac myocytes can be directly affected by the chronic inflammatory processes in HIV infection. Function of the cardiac myocyte is decreased by the chronic inflammation over time, leading to development of myocardial fibrosis.[1] Alterations in the immune system response may trigger autoimmune responses that affect the myocardium, causing myocarditis. Myocardial damage can result from the B-cell stimulation and production of autoantibodies.[1] Damage to the myocardium and conduction system can lead to development of cardiac rhythm disturbances. Cardiac arrhythmias and sudden cardiac death (SCD) are common in HIV infection. Approximately 20% of cardiac deaths in PLWHA are caused by cardiac arrhythmias and SCD.[8] Higher incidence of diastolic dysfunction has been documented in patients infected with HIV who died of SCD compared with patients infected with HIV who died of AIDS-related causes.[20] Both systolic and diastolic dysfunction can occur in HIV infection. However, diastolic dysfunction is more common than systolic dysfunction in HIV-associated cardiomyopathy.[7] Children with HIV infection are also at increased risk of cardiovascular disease, including cardiomyopathy, dyslipidemia, and atherosclerosis.[11]

Pericarditis and pericardial effusion can occur in patients infected with HIV.[8] Pericardial effusions can range from small effusions to effusions large enough to affect cardiac function and cardiac output.[7,21] Pericardial effusions are more common in patients with lower CD4+ cell counts.[7] Patients with lower CD4+ cell counts have a higher incidence of opportunistic infections and malignancies that may directly affect the pericardium. Tuberculosis is an opportunistic infection seen in the HIV population, particularly in developing countries with limited access to cART. Pericardial effusions commonly occur in tuberculosis infections. Tuberculosis must be considered in patients infected with HIV with pericardial effusion, particularly those patients at high risk for opportunistic tuberculosis infections, such as the homeless and individuals in developing countries where access to cART is limited. Pericardial effusions can be moderate to large in patients infected with HIV with an opportunistic tuberculosis infection.[1,8]

PRESENTATION AND CLINICAL ASSESSMENT

Clinical presentation and symptoms associated with cardiovascular disease in patients infected with HIV are similar to those in individuals not infected with HIV.[11] Ischemic cardiovascular conditions seen in PLWHA include ST elevation MI, non–ST elevation MI, acute coronary syndrome (ACS), angina, and silent ischemia.[11] The typical profile of the PLWHA presenting with ACS is a man, aged 50 years or younger, and an ART regimen that includes PIs.[1] Tobacco use and cocaine use have been reported to be more frequent in this group than in patients not infected with HIV.

Individuals with ischemic cardiovascular disease may have chest discomfort, shortness of breath, fatigue, or reduced activity tolerance caused by decreased arterial blood flow to the tissues. Dyspnea with exertion, orthopnea, paroxysmal nocturnal dyspnea, edema, or palpitations may occur in individuals with nonischemic cardiovascular disease. However, HIV-positive patients with ischemia or nonischemic cardiovascular disease are often asymptomatic and may have no symptoms before experiencing a cardiac event.[1,7] It is important for health care professionals to inquire about any symptoms the patient may be experiencing to identify symptoms unrecognized by the patient or symptoms suggestive of underlying cardiovascular disease in this population at high risk for cardiovascular disease and complications.

Complete physical assessment of the cardiovascular system in patients infected with HIV includes collection of subjective and objective data to identify any symptoms; past medical, family, or social history; and physical examination findings that suggest cardiovascular disease. Patients with HIV infection should also be screened for cardiovascular disease with laboratory and diagnostic studies. Documentation of blood pressure recordings, complete lipid profile, and complete metabolic profile to assess for disorders of glucose metabolism, nutritional status, and hepatic and renal function should be included in the patient record.[21]

Traditional cardiovascular risk prediction tools, such as the American College of Cardiology (ACC) and American Heart Association (AHA) Atherosclerotic Cardiovascular Disease risk score and the Framingham Risk Score, have underestimated cardiovascular disease risk in patients with HIV.[24] Diagnostic studies are useful in screening for cardiovascular disease. Twelve-lead electrocardiogram (ECG) and Holter monitor testing can be used to evaluate for arrhythmias. Prolonged QT interval is associated with antiretrovirals and advanced -stage AIDS.[25] Baseline ECG and follow-up ECG can identify conduction abnormalities in advanced-stage disease and treatment.[21] Cardiac enlargement can be seen on standard chest radiograph. Echocardiograms provide information on atrial and ventricular size and function, valvular function and abnormalities, and presence of pericardial effusions.[7] Cardiac MRI may be useful in evaluating cardiac size and function.[8] Coronary computed tomography can be used in evaluation of coronary stenosis as well as plaque morphology for presence of calcification of coronary plaques.[19] Coronary artery calcification and carotid intimal thickness (CIMT) by ultrasonography can be used for evaluation of subclinical atherosclerosis.[16,21,26] Presence of metabolic syndrome is associated with subclinical atherogenesis. Use of PIs in treatment regimens is associated with altered lipid metabolism, fat redistribution (lipodystrophy), and increased risk of metabolic syndrome.[25] CIMT can be used for early detection of subclinical atherogenesis in HIV infection in both adults and children.[26] Cardiac catheterization can be used to define coronary anatomy and further treatment as indicated, including coronary stenting or coronary artery bypass grafting.[1]

TREATMENT

Dyslipidemia is a common problem in PLWHA because of direct effects of HIV viral infection and antiretroviral medication treatment.[21] A complete lipid profile, including total cholesterol, triglycerides, low-density lipoprotein cholesterol, and HDL-C, should be drawn at baseline before initiation of cART and repeated every 3 to 6 months following initiation of treatment.[12]

Lipid level–lowering medications, including statins for cholesterol level reduction and fibrate medications for triglyceride induction, must be initiated appropriately after careful evaluation of risk of potential drug interactions and metabolic considerations. Special consideration for selection of lipid level–lowering therapy must be taken when the patient is also taking PIs.[1] Statin medications used in management of dyslipidemia are commonly metabolized using the cytochrome (CYP) 450 3A4 pathway.[12] PIs can potentiate statin toxicity because of the inhibition effect of these medications on the CYP 450 3A4 pathway.[12] Lipid level–lowering agents that are not metabolized using the CYP 450 pathway should be considered for treatment of dyslipidemia in patients taking PIs. Statin medications that have either no or minimal metabolism via the CYP 450 pathway include pravastatin, rosuvastatin, and pitavastatin. Fenofibrate for treatment of hypertriglyceridemia and ezetimibe for treatment of increased cholesterol levels are nonstatin medications that are not metabolized via the CYP 450 pathway and can be considered for management of dyslipidemia in patients taking PIs.[12]

Management of hypertension and blood pressure monitoring are important to reduce the effect of hypertension on the cardiovascular system. Thiazide diuretics are the first-line therapy for hypertension management in the general population. However, medications such as angiotensin-converting enzyme (ACE) inhibitors are the choice for first-line therapy in PLWHA because of the effect on the renin-angiotensin system for blood pressure control and renal protection.[12]

Anticoagulant medications should be considered in PLWHA just as in the general population with ischemic cardiovascular disease to reduce platelet activity and thrombus formation. Thrombus formation in the setting of coronary and cerebrovascular disease increases the risk of MI or stroke.[1] Aspirin should be considered as an antiplatelet agent unless contraindicated. Potential drug interactions must be evaluated in patients taking PIs and use of other antiplatelet agents commonly used after coronary stenting, such as clopidogrel, prasugrel, and ticagrelor.[1,12]

Management of nonischemic cardiomyopathy in PLWHA includes the use of standard guidelines for heart failure, which includes β-blockers, ACE inhibitors, aldosterone antagonists, and hydralazine-nitrate combination as indicated. Diuretics may be used to manage fluid retention. Special consideration must be given to selection of pharmacologic agents with careful blood pressure monitoring because of possible decreased systemic vascular resistance in advanced illness and potential for hypotension.[8]

RISK FACTORS AND RISK REDUCTION

HIV-positive patients have higher incidences of risk factors associated with cardiovascular disease, including tobacco use, dyslipidemia, metabolic syndrome, and disorders of glucose metabolism and insulin resistance.[12] Cardiovascular risk factor reduction to prevent cardiovascular disease and reduce cardiovascular events is important in the care of PLWHA.[14] Smoking cessation, exercise, and obesity reduction to ideal body weight are important risk factor and lifestyle modifications for PLWHA[8] (Fig. 1).

The incidence of cigarette smoking in PLWHA is 2 to 3 times higher than in the general population.[27] Incidence of cigarette smoking has been reported at between 40% and 70% in PLWHA compared with 19% in the general population.[28] Smoking in PLWHA has been associated with increased respiratory illnesses and cardiovascular disease, lower CD4+ levels, and higher mortality than in nonsmokers.[29] Smoking cessation is an important part of treatment in PLWHA. Use of pharmacologic treatments, including nicotine replacement treatments, antidepressants, and nicotinic receptor agonists that reduce nicotine craving, have been studied in PLWHA. Nonpharmacologic smoking cessation programs using individual or group counseling sessions have also been studied. Combining behavioral counseling with pharmacologic

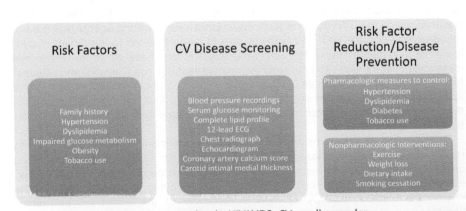

Fig. 1. Cardiovascular health promotion in HIV/AIDS. CV, cardiovascular.

nicotine replacement treatment has been shown to be beneficial for smoking cessation in PLWHA.[29]

Hypertension, dyslipidemia, impaired glucose metabolism, and obesity are common risk factors for cardiovascular disease in PLWHA.[27] Moderate physical exercise has been shown to be beneficial in PLWHA in reduction of waist circumference and weight loss.[6,27] Importance of exercise for weight control and cardiovascular disease prevention should be included in patient education for PLWHA.[21] Dietary education to emphasize the importance of decreased intake of foods high in saturated fat and cholesterol, avoiding foods high in sodium content, and limiting carbohydrate-rich foods can decrease the risk of cardiovascular disease and metabolic syndrome.

SUMMARY

HIV infection is a chronic health condition because of advances in HIV treatment. Life expectancy and risk of cardiovascular disease have increased as a result of treatment advances. Screening for risk and early detection of cardiovascular disease can prevent cardiac-related complications in PLWHA. Treatment strategies to prevent morbidity and mortality from cardiovascular disease complications in PLWHA include pharmacologic and nonpharmacologic measures.

REFERENCES

1. Vachiat A, McCutcheon K, Tsabedze N, et al. HIV and ischemic heart disease. J Am Coll Cardiol 2017;69(1):73–82.
2. World Health Organization. HIV/AIDS fact sheet. Available at: http://www.who.int/mediacentre/factsheets/fs360/en/. Accessed June 1, 2017.
3. Centers for Disease Control and Prevention. HIV/AIDS basic statistics. Available at: https://www.cdc.gov/hiv/basics/statistics.html. Accessed June 1, 2017.
4. McCance KL, Huether SE. Pathophysiology: the biologic basics for disease in adults and children. 7th edition. St Louis (MO): Elsevier; 2014.
5. Shah MR, Cook N, Wong R, et al. Stimulating high impact HIV-related cardiovascular research: recommendations from a multidisciplinary NHLBI working group on HIV-related heart, lung, and blood disease. J Am Coll Cardiol 2015;65(7): 738–44.
6. Conley LJ, Bush TJ, Rupert AW, et al. Obesity is associated with greater inflammation and monocyte activation among HIV-infected adults receiving antiretroviral therapy. AIDS 2015;29:2201–7.
7. Manga P, McCutcheon K, Tsabedze, et al. HIV and nonischemic heart disease. J Am Coll Cardiol 2017;69(1):83–91.
8. Olusegun-Joseph D, Ajuluchukwu J, Okany C, et al. The heart and HIV/AIDS. The Internet Journal of Cardiology 2009;9(1). Available at: http://www.ispub.com/IJC/9/1/7696. Accessed June 1, 2017.
9. Burcham JR, Rosenthal LD. Lehne's pharmacology for nursing care. 9th edition. St Louis (MO): Elsevier; 2016.
10. Hammer GD, McPhee SJ. Pathophysiology of disease: an introduction to clinical medicine. 7th edition. New York: McGraw-Hill; 2014.
11. McDonald CL, Kaltman JR. Cardiovascular disease in adult and pediatric HIV/AIDS. J Am Coll Cardiol 2009;54(13):1185–8.
12. Boccara F, Lang S, Meuleman C, et al. HIV and coronary heart disease. J Am Coll Cardiol 2013;61(5):511–23.

13. Oramasionwu CU, Morse GD, Lawson KA, et al. Hospitalizations for cardiovascular disease in African Americans and whites with HIV/AIDS. Popul Health Manag 2013;16(3):201–7.
14. Lang S, Boccara F, Mary-Krause M, et al. Epidemiology of coronary heart disease in HIV-infected versus uninfected individuals in developed countries. Arch Cardiovasc Dis 2015;108:206–15.
15. Monsuez J, Charniot J, Escaut L, et al. HIV-associated vascular diseases: structural and functional changes, clinical implications. Int J Cardiol 2009;133: 292–306.
16. Krikke M, vanLelyveld SFL, Tesselaar K, et al. The role of T cells in the development of cardiovascular disease in HIV-infected patients. Atherosclerosis 2014; 237:92–8.
17. Escarcega RD, Franco JJ, Mani BC, et al. Cardiovascular disease in patients with chronic human immunodeficiency virus infection. Int J Cardiol 2014;175:1–7.
18. Bittencourt MS, Peixoto D. Atherosclerosis in HIV patients: a different disease or more of the same? Atherosclerosis 2015;240:333–4.
19. D'Ascenzo F, Cerrato E, Calcagno A, et al. High prevalence at computed coronary tomography of non-calcified plaques in asymptomatic HIV patients treated with HAART: a meta-analysis. Atherosclerosis 2015;240:197–204.
20. Secemsky EA, Scherzer R, Nitta E, et al. Novel biomarkers of cardiac stress, cardiovascular dysfunction, and outcomes in HIV-infected individuals. JACC Heart Fail 2015;3(8):591–9.
21. Giannarelli C, Klein RS, Badimon JJ. Cardiovascular implications of HIV-induced dyslipidemia. Atherosclerosis 2011;219:384–9.
22. Strijdom H, Deboever P, Walzl G, et al. Cardiovascular risk and endothelial function in people living with HIV/AIDS: design of the multi-site, longitudinal EndoAfrica study in the Western Cape Province of South Africa. BMC Infect Dis 2017; 17(4):1–9.
23. Jaggers JR, Dudgeon W, Blair SN, et al. A home-based exercise intervention to increase physical activity among people living with HIV: study design of a randomized clinical trial. BMC Public Health 2013;13(502):1–12.
24. Mosepele M, Hemphill LC, Palai T, et al. Cardiovascular disease risk prediction by the American College of Cardiology (ACC)/American Heart Association (AHA) Atherosclerotic Cardiovascular Disease (ASCVD) risk score among HIV-infected patients in sub-Saharan Africa. PLoS One 2017;12(2):e0172897.
25. Fisher SD, Kanda BS, Miller TL, et al. Cardiovascular disease and therapeutic drug-related cardiovascular consequences in HIV-infected patients. Am J Cardiovasc Drugs 2011;11(6):383–94.
26. Alguquerque VM, Zirpoli JC, Mirando-Filho D, et al. Risk factors for subclinical atherosclerosis in HIV-infected patients under and over 40 years: a case-control study. BMC Infect Dis 2013;13(274):1–13.
27. Jaggers JR, Prasad VK, Dudgeon WE, et al. Associations between physical activity and sedentary time on components of metabolic syndrome among adults with HIV. AIDS Care 2014;26(11):1387–92.
28. Balfour L, Wiebe SA, Cameron WD, et al. An HIV-tailored quit-smoking counselling pilot intervention targeting depressive symptoms plus nicotine replacement therapy. AIDS Care 2016;29(1):24–31.
29. Ledgerwood DM, Yskes R. Smoking cessation for people living with HIV/AIDS: a literature review and synthesis. Nicotine Tob Res 2016;18(12):2177–84.

Substance Use Disorders in People Living with Human Immunodeficiency Virus/AIDS

Priyanka Amin, MD[a], Antoine Douaihy, MD[b],*

KEYWORDS

- Substance use disorder • HIV • AIDS • Health outcomes • ART

KEY POINTS

- Existing Data support the high prevalence of the comorbidity of substance use disorder, psychiatric disorder and human immunodeficiency virus illness. Furthermore, there is a vast heterogeneity of people with this "triple diagnosis".
- Each of these comorbidities influences each other, creating a vicious cycle that could potentially result in poor health outcomes.
- An integrated approach to medical, psychiatric, and substance use care provides the best health outcomes.

Substance use disorders (SUDs) and human immunodeficiency virus (HIV) are pervasive overlapping epidemics with a vast array of social and health consequences at individual and societal levels. SUDs are chronic relapsing medical conditions that, if left untreated, result in negative medical, psychological, and social consequences. People who use drugs (PWUD) play a role in the HIV epidemic by simultaneously needing care and potentially transmitting HIV to their injecting and/or sex partners. Therefore, providing effective care to PWUD is essential for both the care of HIV+ individuals as well as the reduction of new diagnoses of HIV. This article covers the prevalence of comorbid SUDs with HIV infection, the complex interactions and impact on negative health outcomes, as well as a practical approach to addressing SUDs in people living with HIV/AIDs (PLWHA).

Disclosure Statement: None (P. Amin). Research support: NIMH (1 RO1 MH109493-01A1), NIDA (U10 DA020036), SAMHSA (1H79T1026446), and Alkermes (6428 A301 and A302). Royalties for 3 academic books from Oxford University Press and PESI Publishing & Media (A. Douaihy).
[a] Department of Psychiatry, Western Psychiatric Institute and Clinic of UPMC, 3811 O'Hara Street, Pittsburgh, PA 15213, USA; [b] Department of Psychiatry, University of Pittsburgh School of Medicine, 3811 O'Hara Street, Pittsburgh, PA 15213, USA
* Corresponding author.
E-mail address: douaihya@upmc.edu

PREVALENCE OF SUBSTANCE USE DISORDERS IN PEOPLE LIVING WITH HUMAN IMMUNODEFICIENCY VIRUS AND AIDS

There are higher rates of substance use among PLWHA than in general populations. Several individuals use more than one drug class, and the overall prevalence of substance use is around 84%.[1] Nicotine use is prevalent in 40% to 70% of individuals in different HIV cohorts.[2] When another substance is used, nicotine use is present in more than 90%. Alcohol is used in 22% to 60% of PLWHA.[3] The prevalence in cocaine use is more variable. Approximately 25% of PWLHA with an alcohol use disorder are also using cocaine.[3] Methamphetamine prevalence rates have not been established. However, methamphetamine use, such as with 3,4-methylenedioxymethamphetamine (MDMA), produces sexual disinhibition and high-risk sexual behavior. The National Survey on Drug Use and Health found that although intravenous (IV) drug users represent 13% of new HIV cases annually, men who have sex with men account for 53% and heterosexual contacts account for 31%.[4] Therefore, drugs, such as MDMA, that increase high-risk sexual behavior significantly contribute to HIV infection.

Triple diagnosis, or the presence of both an SUD and another psychiatric illness along with HIV infection, affected around 10% to 25% of PLWHA.[1] This finding is noteworthy, as individuals with triple diagnosis are more ambivalent about treatment and have increased hopelessness, depression, and suicidality.[1] PLWHA also have higher rates of posttraumatic stress disorder as well as personality disorders, particularly antisocial, avoidant, and borderline personality disorder.[1]

CLINICAL PRESENTATIONS AND MANAGEMENT OF SUBSTANCE INTOXICATION AND WITHDRAWAL

Opioids

The classic description of opioid intoxication is respiratory depression with pinpoint pupils. Other symptoms include bradycardia, hypotension, possible seizures, and coma. The management of clinically significant intoxication, which produces respiratory depression, includes oxygen supplementation and naloxone. Opioid withdrawal symptoms include lacrimation, rhinorrhea, gastrointestinal upset, diarrhea, restlessness, piloerection, muscle and joint aches, and insomnia. Management is symptomatic.

Alcohol and Benzodiazepines

Alcohol intoxication symptoms include slurred speech, gait instability, impaired decision-making, and memory impairment. At high levels of intoxication, somnolence, respiratory depression, coma, and death can occur. Benzodiazepine intoxication symptoms are similar, and benzodiazepines are the first-line treatment of alcohol and benzodiazepine withdrawal. This withdrawal can lead to negative outcomes, including seizures, coma, and death. Individuals without a history of complicated withdrawal can be managed with benzodiazepines as an outpatient through ambulatory detox programs. For people with a history of complicated withdrawal, inpatient management is recommended.

Cocaine

People with cocaine intoxication may presents with hyperthermia, hypertension, tachycardia, tachypnea, and pupillary dilation. They may present with agitation, hypervigilance, and hallucinations. Tremor, diaphoresis, and hyperreflexia may occur. Cocaine intoxication can produce chest pain. Never give beta-blockers for chest pain when it is caused by cocaine. Withdrawal is also managed symptomatically, and generally it does not require any medical intervention.

Methamphetamine

Methamphetamines have both hallucinogenic and stimulant properties. Therefore, the same vital sign changes that occur in cocaine intoxication occur in methamphetamine intoxication. Another finding is nystagmus. Withdrawal symptoms include profound depression, lethargy, increased appetite, and anxiety. Similar to cocaine, management is supportive only. MDMA, known as Molly or ecstasy, is a notable drug that increases empathy, produces euphoria, and heightens senses. The use of MDMA may increase the change of high-risk sexual behavior. In addition, polydipsia may occur and resultant hyponatremia may ensue. Therefore, if individuals who are using MDMA present with an altered mental status, be sure to check their sodium.

COMPLEX INTERACTIONS AND IMPACT LEADING TO ADVERSE HEALTH OUTCOMES

PWUD have increased HIV transmission risk behaviors. Such behaviors include IV drug use with contaminated needles. Acute intoxication, such as with MDMA, increases sexual disinhibition. With a combination of impaired judgment and increased sexual arousal, individuals are more impulsive and are less likely to use condoms or other barriers.

The coexistence of HIV and SUDs is associated with delayed HIV diagnosis and care. PWUDs are less likely to have HIV screening or to have viral load testing. They have less access to and adherence to antiretroviral therapy (ART). Furthermore, they are more likely to have HIV-related symptoms and higher hospitalization rates. PWLHA who are using substances have increased morbidity and mortality, both from HIV and non–HIV-related causes, when compared with PWLHA who are not using substances. For example, people injecting drugs are at an increased risk of infections. Tobacco use is associated with pulmonary infections, oropharyngeal lesions, malignancies, and an increased risk of coronary plaques and heart disease.[2]

Medications that treat SUDs often interact with ARTs, resulting in altered concentrations of ARTs and/or medications. This interplay may lead to opioid withdrawal symptoms, which place individuals at risk for relapse, opioid withdrawal symptoms, or insufficient dosing of ARTs. This subject is explored in more detail later in this article.

AIDS-related events are no longer the major causes of death for PLWHA after the introduction of ARTs. PLWHA are now dying of the same causes as the general population. For example, smoking nicotine leads to an increase in coronary heart disease, bone disease and fractures, and infections, such as pneumonia.[2] Smoking undermines the life expectancy of PLWHA on ART more than the HIV infection does. This discrepancy grows more pronounced with increasing age.[2]

The treatment of substance use is effective in decreasing the aforementioned disparities in PLWHA who also have a SUD. For example, smoking cessation leads to decreased health problems associated with HIV infections after 3 months of abstinence, with the combination of nicotine replacement therapy (NRT) and counseling. The incidence of pneumonia decreases. Individuals also have decreased use of other substances, such as cocaine.

However, a provider barrier to addressing tobacco use is that smoking cessation is often not perceived as a high priority in the treatment of PLWHA. Providers may have the false notion that the negative impacts of smoking are not as deleterious as those of HIV infection. They may also think individuals do not want to stop smoking. However, more than half of PLWHA who smoke cigarettes have contemplated smoking cessation, and more than half have tried to stop at least once. Predictors of smoking cessation success include a high level of motivation to stop and a low degree of dependence. Therefore, counseling and brief interventions, such as motivational interviewing, can be helpful in guiding patients through the stages of behavioral change and in strengthening motivation to stop tobacco use. Dependence can be decreased through NRT and through other medication assistance, such as bupropion and varenicline.

APPROACH TO TREATMENT OF PEOPLE LIVING WITH HUMAN IMMUNODEFICIENCY VIRUS AND AIDS WITH CO-OCCURRING SUBSTANCE USE DISORDERS
Seek, Test, Treat, and Retain

The goal is to seek, test, treat, and retain PLWHA and SUDs in substance use treatment and foster adherence to ART and medical treatment (**Fig. 1**).

About one in 5 individuals with HIV are undiagnosed, and many of these people have SUDs.[4] Therefore, offering HIV testing in substance use treatment as well as in jails, prisons, and emergency departments (EDs) where individuals with SUDs may also end up can help identify people with HIV.

Once someone has been identified with HIV, linkage to treatment should be prompt. Barriers to treatment include younger age, female sex, unstable housing, low socioeconomic status, lack of insurance, and lower health literacy. Personal attitudes and preference to defer treatment also delays treatment.[5] For example, an individual who is not experiencing symptoms from HIV may not think they need treatment. Of note, clinicians also delay treatment because of their beliefs that treating HIV in individuals with SUDs may be futile or their attitude that they would rather not treat people with SUDs at all.[5] People with SUDs may have interruptions in care if incarcerated, such as for drug-related charges.

Some of the ways to decrease these barriers and improve treatment compliance include giving people take-home naloxone (Narcan) in the event of an opioid overdose. Also, neurocognitive impairment and intoxication make it more challenging to adhere to medication regimens. Therefore, providing pillboxes for patients, helping them set alarms in their phone for when to take medication, or offering directly administered ART (DAART) may improve adherence. DAART could include mobile programs with home visits. Lastly, intensive case management may be helpful to coordinate care for PLWHA who have SUDs. Unfortunately, retention, measured nationally by attending a clinic with laboratory monitoring quarterly, is only about 50% in PLWHA and is lower with comorbid SUDs; with IV drug use, retention is even lower.[5] Therefore, international guidelines recommend integrated care. If an integrated treatment approach is not feasible, then actively screen for substance use and make referrals for treatment.

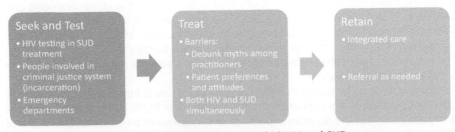

Fig. 1. Seek, test, treat, and retain model for comorbid HIV and SUD.

Integrated Care

Both HIV and SUDs are chronic illnesses that fluctuate in severity and activity over time, and they have complex interactions that translate into worse health outcomes. Identifying substance use is important, yet providers do not sufficiently screen for this. In a sample of almost 1000 HIV+ adults, 71% were using substances, less than 50% had discussed substance use with their HIV treatment provider, and only 24% were in substance use treatment.[5] Treating underlying substance use increases HIV treatment and decreases the risk of HIV seroconversion. In one study, for individuals who use IV heroin, after 18 months, 22.0% of them became HIV+ when getting treatment as usual versus 3.5% of those on methadone.[6] Given that methadone is only available at methadone clinics, previously, providers were unable to provide medication-assisted treatment of opioid use disorder. However, this changed with buprenorphine.

Buprenorphine is supplied either alone (eg, Subutex) or in combination with naloxone (eg, Suboxone). The naloxone prevents individuals from achieving a high by snorting or injecting buprenorphine. Buprenorphine is different from methadone in that it is a partial agonist instead of a full agonist at the mu receptor. As such, it is something that does not require patients to go to a special clinic. Rather, physicians can prescribe this after an 8-hour training and an application for extension of their Drug Enforcement Administration license to include Suboxone. This accessibility has made it easier to have integrated care for PLWHA, as any physician can become a prescriber.

Integrated treatment (**Fig. 2**) is crucial for ensuring access to ART and substance use treatment as well as for providing people with SUDs access to HIV treatment. A

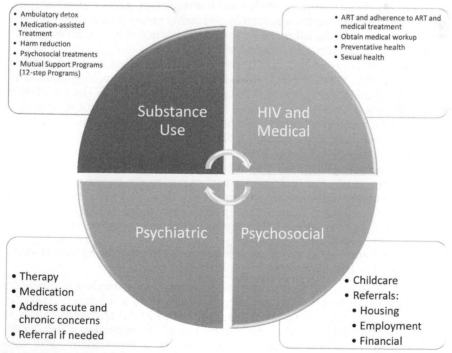

- Ambulatory detox
- Medication-assisted Treatment
- Harm reduction
- Psychosocial treatments
- Mutual Support Programs (12-step Programs)

- ART and adherence to ART and medical treatment
- Obtain medical workup
- Preventative health
- Sexual health

Substance Use

HIV and Medical

Psychiatric

Psychosocial

- Therapy
- Medication
- Address acute and chronic concerns
- Referral if needed

- Childcare
- Referrals:
  - Housing
  - Employment
  - Financial

Fig. 2. The integrated care model.

barrier to this integration is the myth that PWUDs will be noncompliant with ARTs and, thus, treatment would be futile.[7] Perpetuation of this myth will result in more individuals with SUDs seroconverting to being HIV+, will continue to delay diagnosis and treatment, and will result in increased morbidity and mortality that could have been prevented.

Integrated care models should address substance use, psychiatric symptoms, HIV and other medical comorbidities, and psychosocial needs.

Substance use management in clinical settings would ideally involve ambulatory detox from substances, pharmacologic treatment of SUDs, and harm-reduction approaches. Individuals who are withdrawing from alcohol or benzodiazepines who do not have a history of complicated withdrawal (eg, no prior withdrawal-related seizures) as well as individuals withdrawing from opioids are appropriate for ambulatory detox. Pharmacologic treatment of SUDs for providers caring for PLWHA includes buprenorphine for opioid use disorder as well as other medications. Additional details regarding pharmacologic treatment are discussed later in this section. Harm reduction for SUDs would include providing naloxone to PWUDs in case of opioid overdose, a needle exchange program for individuals who inject drugs, as well as barrier methods for sexual intercourse, such as condoms. If possible, group meetings, such as Alcoholics Anonymous/Narcotics Anonymous or skill-building/therapy groups, can also be helpful for the treatment of SUDs; these could be offered either within the clinic or through informing interested individuals about these groups.

Psychiatric management should address both acute and chronic mental health symptoms through both therapy and pharmacologic management. If a clinic is unable to provide these resources, then having a list of referrals for patients and ensuring they can access options is appropriate.

For HIV and medical management, clinics should provide medications, obtain laboratory test results as indicated, monitor and manage other medical conditions, and engage in preventative health care, such as discussing smoking cessation. Providers can address sexual risk by asking about sexual behaviors and having access to barriers, such as free condoms available at the clinic.

In addition, clinical settings should address psychosocial concerns and patients' needs. For example, to help parents, ideally clinics would have caregiving capabilities, such as a lactation room or a daycare that parents could have their children at while they see their care providers and receive treatment. People with SUDs often have chaotic lifestyles that may be complicated by limited finances, homelessness, and unemployment. Therefore, other considerations for an integrated health clinic include providing individuals with housing, financial, and occupational resources.

The risk of not having integrated care that addresses all of the aforementioned components, substance use, HIV, and other medical, mental health, and psychosocial concerns, is that more individuals will be lost to treatment. There is a frequent dropout rate of treatment due to worsening substance use, psychiatric illness, psychosocial stressors, and/or health. Therefore, this model is crucial to retaining individuals in treatment.

Medication Management of Substance Use Disorders in People Living with Human Immunodeficiency Virus and AIDS

For opioid use disorder, medication-assisted treatment with methadone or buprenorphine is an effective treatment in decreasing the relapse rate and duration of relapse.

Methadone has several drug-drug interactions with ARTs. Methadone leads to increased zidovudine levels, which can become toxic, so monitoring is recommended.[5,8] Opioid withdrawal is common for people on methadone who take non-nucleoside reverse transcriptase inhibitors, such as efavirenz or nevirapine.[8]

Clinicians should also monitor for withdrawal symptoms when starting rilpivirine. For individuals on methadone, a higher dose may be required if taking protease inhibitors, specifically lopinavir, ritonavir, or tipranavir.[8] Although nelfinavir does decrease the area under curve (AUC) for methadone, clinically this has not been shown to lead to withdrawal or require a dose adjustment.[8] Methadone also has interactions with commonly prescribed antibiotics. Fluconazole increases the level of methadone, whereas rifampin can precipitate withdrawal from methadone.[5]

Buprenorphine has few drug-drug interactions. The one exception is atazanavir, which increases buprenorphine's area under the curve and may have oversedation.[8] Additionally, atazanavir must be boosted with ritonavir for people on buprenorphine.[5,8]

Integrase inhibitors have had no effects on methadone or buprenorphine, or vice versa, based on clinical trials.[8] There is a lack of research on C-C chemokine receptor type 5 (CCR5; maraviroc) antagonists and their interactions with methadone and buprenorphine.

Naltrexone in oral form (ReVia) and extended-release injectable form (Vivitrol) is another treatment of opioid use disorder as well as other SUDs, such as alcohol use disorder. It is an effective treatment with highly motivated individuals. There are no known interactions with ART, as this has not been studied.[5] For alcohol use disorder, naltrexone increases the time to relapse and to decrease the number of heavy drinking days that patients have.[5]

There are 2 other medications for alcohol use disorder: acamprosate (Campral) and disulfiram. Acamprosate is dosed 3 times a day, so adherence presents a challenge. Acamprosate increases abstinence from alcohol, though there is no difference in relapse rates.[5] Disulfiram is an aversion therapy, as it causes patients to feel ill when they drink alcohol. Disulfiram should not be given with amprenavir or metronidazole.[5] It can be used for motivated patients in conjunction with other therapies.

NRT does not seem to interfere with ART. However, NRT is not as effective in smoking cessation as other medications, such as varenicline (Chantix) and bupropion (Zyban). Varenicline is dosed twice daily, and the cost may be prohibitive for patients. In early studies, there were no interactions with ART.[5] Varenicline has the highest rates of abstinence from and reductions in smoking. Furthermore, it has been shown to increase the CD4 count.[5] Bupropion is also quite effective, particularly when used in conjunction with other therapies. Two medications that decrease bupropion concentrations are efavirenz and lopinavir.[5]

For crack cocaine, lamotrigine can be useful and given to individuals with HIV. For methamphetamine use, naltrexone and mirtazapine can be helpful as well.

Addressing Health Care Practitioners' Misperceptions and the Righting Reflex

Practitioners have misperceptions regarding comorbid SUD and HIV infection. For example, a common myth is that people who use IV drugs will have higher rates of ART resistance. In actuality, both groups have similar ART resistance rates. Health care practitioners may also think that they must treat SUDs first, with an individual being abstinent for some period, before the initiation of ART. However, this leads to a delay in care; there is no absolute contraindication in the treatment of HIV in people with SUDs. On the other hand, there are those who think tobacco use is not as important to address during visits. However, as previously discussed in this article, PLWHA are more likely to have morbidity and mortality due to smoking-associated illnesses than primary HIV/AIDS. Therefore, providers cannot overlook the importance of preventative health in caring for PLWHA.

One of the barriers people working with individuals with SUDs have is the "righting reflex," which is the "desire to fix," as outlined in motivational interviewing.[9] This reflex is often not consciously recognized and involves clinicians feeling like they need to "make things right." Although the reflex may not seem problematic on the surface, it leads to a decrease in patient autonomy and can lead to practitioners' burnout.

CASE DISCUSSION

A 44-year-old married African American man with a recent diagnosis of HIV, chronic anemia, traumatic brain injury, depression, and alcohol and opioid use disorders presented to the ED after a suicide attempt via an overdose on oxycodone.

The patient has been known to the hospital system for more than a year, presenting to the ED for various complaints, including shortness of breath, dyspnea on exertion, lethargy, and dysphagia. At each visit, it was noted that the patient had severe anemia, requiring multiple transfusions, and leukopenia. Several possible diagnoses were evaluated, including occult malignancy; however, HIV was never considered in the differential, and the patient was not tested during these ED visits. The progression of his symptoms led to disability and loss of his job. Perceiving that he could not adequately provide for his family, he started experiencing depressive symptoms and suicidal ideation for the first time with intent but no plan. Consequently, he required inpatient psychiatric hospitalization for 3 days. He was discharged with a prescription for citalopram but was not adherent with it or outpatient psychiatric treatment.

Several months later, the patient presented to the ED with nausea, vomiting, and recurrent dysphagia and was found to have appendicitis. In light of his leukopenia and likely esophageal candidiasis, an HIV test was performed. He was then informed that he has full-blown AIDS, with a total CD4 count of 3 cells per cubic millimeter. Of note, the patient reports being monogamous with his wife of 4 years, who tested negative for HIV. The patient had an appendectomy and was discharged home. He did not follow up with medical treatment at the HIV clinic; therefore, he was never started on ART. He returned to the hospital; this time it was for his mother, to whom he was very close. She died a day later.

Two months later, he started experiencing severe clinical depression mixed with grief related to the loss of his mother. He reported that he felt hopeless and started to have thoughts that he wished to be with her. He had a fifth of vodka and ingested 30 pills of oxycodone and called his sister to say goodbye, leading to inpatient hospitalization on the dual-diagnosis unit.

The case demonstrates 2 important aspects of fighting the HIV epidemic: the utility of universal screening and strategies to address comorbid psychiatric and SUDs. The patient's late HIV diagnosis, depression, and alcohol and opioid use disorders are intertwined and played important roles in his overall clinical presentations; but their exact relationship remains unclear. Did the patient's alcohol and opioid use lead to risky sexual behaviors and contracting HIV? Did a preexisting mood disorder contribute to alcohol and opioid use and suicidality? Did coping with HIV illness and grief compound an alcohol and opioid use disorder to acutely worsen his depression? Providing an integrated approach to medical, psychiatric, and substance use care can result in optimizing clinical outcomes.

REFERENCES

1. Durvasula R, Miller TR. Substance abuse treatment in persons with HIV/AIDS: challenges in managing triple diagnosis. Behav Med 2014;40(2):43–52.

2. Calvo M, Laguno M, Martinez M, et al. Effects of tobacco smoking on HIV-infected individuals. AIDS Rev 2015;17:47–55.

3. International AIDS Society-USA. Substance use disorders in HIV-infected patients: impact and new treatment strategies. Top HIV Med 2004;12(3):77–82.
4. Substance Abuse and Mental Health Services Administration, Center for Behavioral Health Statistics and Quality. The NSDUH report: HIV/AIDS and substance use. Rockville (MD): 2010. Available at: http://archive.samhsa.gov/data/2k10/HIV-AIDS/HIV-AIDs.htm. Accessed July 12, 2017.
5. Meyer JP, Althoff AL, Altice FL. Optimizing care for HIV-infected people who use drugs: evidence-based approaches to overcoming healthcare disparities. Clin Infect Dis 2013;57:1309–17.
6. Metzger DS, Woody GE, McLellan AT, et al. Human immunodeficiency virus seroconversion among intravenous drug users in and out-of-treatment: an 18-month prospective follow-up. J Acquir Immune Defic Syndr 1993;6:1049–56.
7. Korthuis PT, Josephs JS, Fleishman JA, et al. Substance abuse treatment in human immunodeficiency virus: the role of patient–provider discussions. J Subst Abuse Treat 2008;35(3):294–303.
8. Bruce RD, Moody DE, Altice FL, et al. A review of pharmacological interactions between HIV or HCV medications and opioid agonist therapy: implications and management for clinical practice. Expert Rev Clin Pharmacol 2013;6(3):249–69.
9. Miller WR, Rollnick S. Motivational interviewing: helping people change. 3rd edition. New York: Guilford Press; 2013.

FURTHER READING

Volkow ND, Montaner J. The urgency of providing comprehensive and integrated treatment for substance abusers with HIV. Health Aff (Millwood) 2011;30(8): 1411–9.

Best Practices and Self-Care to Support Women in Living Well with Human Immunodeficiency Virus/AIDS

Melinda Ann Bogardus, RN, MSN, FNP-BC[a,b,c],*

KEYWORDS

- HIV positive • Women • Gender inequality • Substance abuse • Violence
- Depression • Best practices • Self-care

KEY POINTS

- Human immunodeficiency virus (HIV) infection among women in the United States has declined overall but is still a formidable health problem, disproportionately affecting the most vulnerable women.
- African American, Latino, and other racial/ethnic minority women bear the greatest burden of HIV/AIDS in the United States.
- The higher prevalence of HIV in US black and Latino communities accounts for the disproportionate incidence of this infection in black and Latino women.
- Challenges faced more often by HIV-positive women include poverty, poor-quality education, depression, and trauma.
- Psychosocial assessments and interventions are fundamental to the overall care and promotion of health in HIV-positive women.

INTRODUCTION

This article highlights characteristics and needs of human immunodeficiency virus (HIV)-positive women in the United States and discusses best practices and self-care to achieve optimal health in this population. In particular, the article focuses on racial and ethnic minority women and women experiencing challenges known to be

The author has no commercial or financial conflicts of interest to disclose and has received no funding from any source for this work.
[a] Walden University, College of Health Sciences, School of Nursing, 100 Washington Avenue South, Suite 900, Minneapolis, MN 55401, USA; [b] East Tennessee State University, College of Nursing, 365 Stout Drive, Johnson City, TN 37614, USA; [c] AppHealthCare, Ashe Health Center, 413 McConnell Street, Jefferson, NC 28640, USA
* Corresponding author. 278 Sunset Mountain Road, Boone, NC 28607.
E-mail address: melinda.bogardus2@waldenu.edu

Nurs Clin N Am 53 (2018) 67–82
https://doi.org/10.1016/j.cnur.2017.10.008
0029-6465/18/© 2017 Elsevier Inc. All rights reserved.

nursing.theclinics.com

social determinants of health, that is, poverty, lack of insurance, poor-quality education, homelessness, substance abuse, violence, and discrimination, because such women are disproportionately affected by HIV. It is important to develop not only gender-appropriate but also culturally competent care when partnering with HIV-positive women.[1]

Human Immunodeficiency Virus/AIDS in United States Women

The incidence of HIV infection for women in the United States was initially low, increased dramatically during the late 1980s, peaked in the early 1990s, and began to decline several years into the 2000s[2,3] (**Fig. 1**). From 2005 to 2014, the incidence of HIV in this group dropped by 40%.[4] The total number of HIV-positive women in the United States by the end of 2014 was 230,360[5] and, in 2015, women accounted for 19% of new HIV infections and 24% of new AIDS diagnoses.[2,5] Of the 1,216,917 cumulative AIDS cases in the United States, women make up 20% or 248,270.[2]

Rates of HIV/AIDS in US women clearly demonstrate racial and ethnic disparities. African American women bear the heaviest burden of new and existing HIV/AIDS diagnoses. Their rates per 100,000 for new HIV and AIDS diagnoses were 26.2 and 16.2 in 2015 compared with 1.6 and 0.9 for non-Latino white women.[5] Black women represented 60% of all US women living with HIV as recently as 2014 and accounted for 64% of new HIV infections in women in 2015.[2,6,7] Although Latina women have HIV/AIDS rates far below those of African American women,[5] this group has also been disproportionately affected. Latinas had 4 times the likelihood of being diagnosed with HIV compared with non-Latino white women by 2013[3] and, at the end of 2014, represented 17% of HIV-positive women in the United States.[2] Like African American and Latino women, women from other minority groups living in the United States had higher rates of new HIV/AIDS diagnoses in 2015 than non-Latino white women[5] (**Table 1**).

Why Are Minority Women Affected More by Human Immunodeficiency Virus?

That black, Latina, and some other racial/ethnic minority women in the United States have been disproportionately affected by HIV/AIDS does not mean they engage in higher-risk activities than non-Latino white women.[3] What explains their higher rates of HIV infection is that they choose partners (either sexual, drug use, or both) largely from their own racial and ethnic communities that have higher prevalence of HIV; thus, these women are more likely than non-Latino white women to be exposed to HIV.[2,3,8]

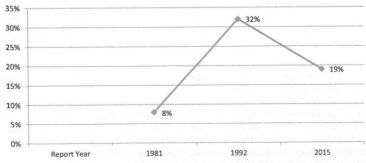

Fig. 1. Incidence of HIV in US women. (*Data from* The Henry J. Kaiser Family Foundation. A report on women and HIV/AIDS in the United States 2013. Available at: http://www.womenhiv.org/wp-content/uploads/2013/06/KFF-2013-report-on-women-and-HIV.pdf. Accessed June 12, 2017.)

Table 1
Incidence of human immunodeficiency virus/AIDS diagnosis in women by race/ethnicity (2015)

African American HIV/AIDS Number (Rate per 100,000)	Latina HIV/AIDS Number (Rate per 100,000)	Asian HIV/AIDS Number (Rate per 100,000)	American Indian/ Alaska Native HIV/AIDS Number (Rate per 100,000)	Native Hawaiian/ Other Pacific Islander HIV/AIDS Number (Rate per 100,000)	Multiple Races HIV/ AIDS Number (Rate per 100,000)	White HIV/AIDS Number (Rate per 100,000)	All Women HIV/ AIDS Number (Rate per 100,000)
4524 (26.2)/ 2804 (16.2)	1131 (5.3)/ 632 (2.9)	132 (1.7)/52 (0.7)	55 (5.6)/39 (4.0)	8 (3.5)/3 (1.3)	121 (5.5)/164 (7.5)	1431 (1.6)/ 765 (0.9)	7402 (5.4)/ 4459 (3.2)

Adapted from The Centers for Disease Control and Prevention (CDC). HIV surveillance report, 2015. Available at: http://www.cdc.gov/hiv/library/reports/hiv-surveillance.html. Accessed June 5, 2017.

Greater stigma around homosexuality/bisexuality in the black and Latino communities compared with that in the White community has contributed to the former communities' less-effective HIV prevention efforts and higher HIV prevalence.[8,9] To provide some perspective on HIV disparity in the United States, consider that in 2015, blacks comprised 13.3% of the population but accounted for 45% of new HIV infections, and Latinos made up 17.6% of the population and represented 23% of new infections.[5,10] By contrast, non-Latino whites comprised 77.1% of the population and only 27% of new HIV diagnoses.[5,10]

Human Immunodeficiency Virus Care, Antiretroviral Treatment, and Virus Suppression in United States Women

In 2014, 76% of HIV-positive women accessed health care within 1 month of their diagnosis.[2] At the end of 2013, rates of retention in HIV care and HIV viral load suppression for women diagnosed in 2012 or earlier were 57% and 52%, respectively.[2] Other Centers for Disease Control and Prevention data on HIV-positive women revealed that, as of 2012, 85% knew their HIV status and 70% were linked to HIV medical care, but only 41% remained in care and, of the 36% who received prescriptions for antiretroviral treatment (ART), just 26% were virally suppressed.[11] Viral suppression across groups of women shows yet another racial and ethnic disparity with regard to HIV with rates of 21% for African American women, 26% for Latinas, and 30% for non-Latino white women.[12] All these rates fall well below the National HIV/AIDS Strategy's goal of viral load suppression in at least 80% of patients.[13]

Mortality in United States Women with Human Immunodeficiency Virus/AIDS

There were 6721 deaths of men and women in the United States in 2014 due to HIV.[4] Women accounted for 1783 or 27% of this total,[2] a proportion exceeding their 2014 HIV prevalence of 24%.[5] Untreated HIV-positive women appear to die 5 to 10 years earlier than untreated HIV-positive men.[14] Although not among the top 10 causes of death for most US women in 2014, HIV was the fourth, sixth, and seventh leading cause of death for African American women aged 35 to 44, 25 to 34, and 20 to 24, respectively.[15]

Modes of Transmission for Women in the United States with Human Immunodeficiency Virus/AIDS

Since the mid-1990s, heterosexual activity has been the dominant mode of HIV transmission for women.[3] Before that, it was injection drug use (IDU).[3] Heterosexual transmission accounted for 86% or 6392 of the 7402 new HIV infections in US women in 2015.[2,5] IDU accounted for 980 and other risk, that is, hemophilia, blood transfusion, perinatal exposure, and risk factor not reported, accounted for 32 of these new infections.[5] Non-Latino white women had the highest rate of HIV due to IDU in 2015[2] (**Table 2**).

CHARACTERISTICS AND EXPERIENCES OF WOMEN WITH HUMAN IMMUNODEFICIENCY VIRUS/AIDS
Socioeconomic, Demographic, and Geographic Characteristics

HIV-positive women in the United States come disproportionately from communities of color. Although this disease affects women from all socioeconomic statuses in this country, HIV-positive women are more likely than uninfected women and HIV-positive men to live in poverty.[1,16] Women with HIV also often lack transportation; reside in communities with high rates of HIV, sexually transmitted diseases (STDs), incarceration, and violence; and many are primary caregivers of children and others.[1,16–20]

Table 2
Number of human immunodeficiency virus/AIDS diagnoses in women by race/ethnicity and transmission category (2015)

	African American	Latina	Asian	American Indian/ Alaska Native	Native Hawaiian/ Other Pacific Islander	Multiple Races	White	All Women
Heterosexual contact	4142/2423	1010/487	125/47	40/28	6/2	100/109	968/496	6391/3592
IDU	363/339	115/121	6/3	15/11	2/1	20/49	458/260	980/786
Other	19/42	5/24	0/2	0/0	0/0	1/5	5/9	31/82

Adapted from The Centers for Disease Control and Prevention (CDC). HIV surveillance report, 2015. Available at: http://www.cdc.gov/hiv/library/reports/hiv-surveillance.html. Accessed June 5, 2017.

Although most US women with HIV are young and of reproductive age, because of treatment advances and more universal screening practices, the number of older women living or newly diagnosed with HIV has grown.[14] Older individuals get diagnosed with HIV later and have greater mortality.[14] As HIV affects women of all ages, it is important for their health providers to be aware of key contraceptive, preconception, prenatal and postpartum, gynecologic, and postmenopausal women's health issues.

Most diagnoses of HIV in the United States concentrate in urban areas except in the South.[6,21] According to a report funded by the Henry J. Kaiser Family Foundation,[3] the highest prevalence of HIV infection in women as of 2013 was in 3 areas: the South, the Northeast, and Washington, DC. Analysis of more recent data from state and local health departments revealed that the US counties with the highest prevalence of HIV in women relative to men were the most socioeconomically disadvantaged counties in the Deep South[22] (**Fig. 2**).

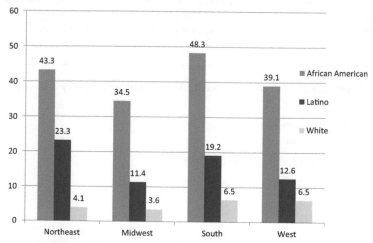

Fig. 2. Rates per 100,000 of HIV by race/ethnicity and geographic region. (*Data from* Centers for Disease Control and Prevention (CDC). HIV surveillance report, 2015. Available at: http://www.cdc.gov/hiv/library/reports/hiv-surveillance.html. Accessed June 5, 2017.)

Experience of Human Immunodeficiency Virus/AIDS Stigma

Stigma, a feeling or experience of being labeled as socially deviant or disgraceful, surrounds conditions like HIV/AIDS.[20] Stigma can have uniquely negative impacts on HIV-positive women.[19,20] Taylor[20] found that women experiencing HIV stigma prioritized the health of their children and others over their own and avoided disclosure and addressing their health needs because of fears of being denied services, being ostracized, and/or having their children taken from them. HIV-positive women reported to Squires and colleagues[19] that their health care providers often failed to discuss family planning, preconception health, and pregnancy. This gap in care suggested disapproval on the part of health care providers of HIV-positive women having sexual and reproductive lives. Fifty-nine percent of this sample thought that society disapproved of HIV-positive women reproducing.[19]

Health-Related Experiences of Human Immunodeficiency Virus–Positive Women

Compared with HIV-positive men, HIV-positive women generally have more negative health care and health experiences (**Box 1**); in addition, they are more psychologically and physiologically vulnerable because of sex- and gender-related stressors (eg, reproductive decisions, caregiver burden, and intimate partner violence [IPV]).[16,23,24] Armas-Kolostroubis and Cheever[25] reported that HIV-positive women may be less likely to keep their initial appointment, remain in care, and adhere to ART. Possible explanations for these findings, other than women prioritizing others' needs over their own, include having more ART side effects; being more susceptible to psychological problems; having experiences of past or on-going violence; having more frequent homelessness; and/or having greater guilt and worry about the impact of HIV on children.[25]

Psychosocial Characteristics and Challenges of Human Immunodeficiency Virus–Positive Women

Women generally have less power in society and relationships and thus less control over their lives and sexuality.[1,14,26] Gender inequality, which is exacerbated by the intersection of marginalizing identities of race, culture, and class, can negatively influence the experiences of HIV-positive women.[1,26] HIV-positive women are more likely than HIV-negative women to report psychosocial problems, including past or current substance use/abuse, violence, and depression or other mental illness.[19,27,28]

Box 1
Negative health care and health experiences of human immunodeficiency virus–positive women

Receive their HIV diagnosis later

Receive lower quality care

Rely more on publically funded health coverage

Prescribed less effective ART

Have poorer health

Have more hospitalizations

Are recruited less often into HIV clinical trials

Data from US Department of Health and Human Services, Health Resources and Services Administration. A guide to the clinical care of women with HIV. Rockville (MD): US DHHS; 2013.

Substance use/abuse

Alcohol and illicit substance abuse rates of 8% and 33%, respectively, have been reported for persons with HIV in the United States.[12] Data from the Women's Interagency HIV Study (WIHS) (N = 2058) revealed a prevalence of crack or cocaine use or IDU of 27%.[26] Another more recent study of HIV-positive women (N = 138) found that 76.8% of the sample had a history of either alcohol or illicit substance abuse.[29]

Whether substance abuse begins or increases after HIV diagnosis, addiction can compromise a woman's health. Time, energy, and money may largely be spent on procuring and ingesting drugs with little of these resources remaining for self-care.[26] Substance abuse can interfere with both being prescribed and adhering well to ART.[26] Women abusing substances may take more sexual and drug use risks, increasing their likelihood of HIV reinfection (with the consequences of acquiring different and resistant strains of HIV and increasing viral load) and infection with other diseases harmful to their health. Finally, women addicted to alcohol or drugs may have decreased agency to leave violent relationships and are more vulnerable to mental health problems.[26]

Violence

HIV-positive and -negative women with comparable sociodemographic backgrounds have reported similar rates of violence, but HIV-positive women may experience violence more often and severely.[26,30] Others have argued that HIV-positive women have rates of violence twice those of uninfected women.[31] A meta-analysis (N = 5930) on psychological trauma in HIV-positive women found the following rates of violence: 55.3% for IPV, 61.1% for lifetime sexual abuse, and 72.1% for lifetime physical abuse.[31] A survey study of 113 HIV-positive women revealed lifetime history of trauma and coerced sexual activity rates of 71.8% and 64.5%, respectively.[32] Rates of sexual abuse, physical abuse, and domestic violence of 55%, 75%, and 62%, respectively, were calculated in yet another sample of HIV-positive women.[29]

It has been speculated that violence against women may increase with disclosure of their HIV status and with attempting to negotiate condom use.[33,34] Reported rates of violence against women associated with disclosure range from 0.5% to 4%,[33,34] and there is no evidence that negotiating condom use increases violence.[34] Nevertheless, several experts advise assessing the potential for violence before recommending these actions to women.[26,33,34]

Mental health problems

Depression is the most common mental health problem in HIV-positive women.[26] The prevalence of chronic depressive symptoms in women in the HIV Epidemiology Research Study (N = 765) and the WIHS (N = 2058) was 43% and 50%, respectively.[19] Two more recent studies on HIV-positive women found 27% endorsing 5 or more symptoms of depression[19] and 47.7% reporting depression.[32] Overall, research has demonstrated HIV-positive women to have twice the rate of depression of uninfected women and consistently higher rates of depression than men with HIV.[17,19,28] Chronic depression with HIV has been shown to correlate with decreased immune function, more rapid progression of HIV disease,[17] and increased mortality.[1,19,26]

BEST PRACTICES IN CARING FOR WOMEN WITH HUMAN IMMUNODEFICIENCY VIRUS/AIDS

General Medical Care of Human Immunodeficiency Virus–Positive Women

For a comprehensive overview of the care of HIV-positive women, it is recommended to consult the US Department of Health and Human Services (DHHS) publication, *A Guide to the Clinical Care of Women with HIV,*[16] and to visit the US DHHS Health

Resources and Services Administration Web site for updates. This section strives to highlight clinical care issues most pertinent to HIV-positive women rather than covering all aspects of general HIV medical care.

HIV-positive women need high-quality medical care that is confidential, nonjudgmental, holistic, patient centered, and, if possible, team based.[23] The frequency of medical visits will depend upon numerous factors.[29] Ideally, when initiating HIV care in women, frequent, closely spaced visits should be scheduled in order to gain their trust; help them adjust to their diagnosis; allow sufficient time to sensitively explore and address mental health, current or past violence, and substance use issues; and create a safe environment so that procedures like a Papanicolaou (Pap) test and pelvic examination are not traumatic.[23]

HIV-positive women will likely need gynecologic and, in many cases, obstetric specialty care. These providers should either themselves be experienced in HIV or work closely with HIV medicine specialists. Other important care team members who ideally should be integrated within HIV medical services include nurses, pharmacists, behavioral health providers, social workers, case managers, and peer counselors.[23]

Sexual and Reproductive Health Needs

Health professionals of HIV-positive women should be proactive and nonjudgmental in assessing and addressing sexual and reproductive health needs.[19,23,26,35] They should ask women about sexual practices, number and sex of partners, sexual partners' risk activities, STD diagnoses and symptoms, condom and contraceptive use and preferences, symptoms of sexual dysfunction, and future reproductive plans.[19,23,26,35] In discussing these topics sensitively and openly, health care providers can help reduce stigma as well as incidence of STDs, HIV reinfection, and unplanned pregnancies.

Antiretroviral Treatment and Women with Human Immunodeficiency Virus

Women should be prescribed the most practical, well-tolerated, and effective ART as soon after their diagnosis as possible.[25,35–37] For the most current recommendations on ART for women, 2 different sets of guidelines may be consulted: the DHHS ART guidelines for adults and adolescents[36] and those for pregnant women.[37]

On entry into HIV or prenatal care, before starting ART, and whenever there is suboptimal HIV viral suppression on ART, nonjudgmental assessment of potential or actual ART adherence should occur.[25,36,37] The latter assessment should explore adherence barriers (**Box 2**).[26] Before prescribing ART, health care providers should explain how it works, the treatment goals, and the rationale for 95% or better adherence.[25] Anticipatory guidance about possible side effects and adverse reactions is crucial.[25] Finally, health care providers should seek to understand and respond to any fears or doubts patients may have with regard to taking ART.[25]

Different pharmacokinetics and adverse effects of antiretroviral treatment in women

Although ART has been shown to be effective in controlling HIV in women, it is important to explain that most clinical trials studying the pharmacologic activity, efficacy, and safety of ART have involved men.[19] The pharmacokinetics of some antiretroviral medications in women may not mirror those in men because of physiologic differences such as in plasma volume and cytochrome P450 function.[36] Women may have increased frequency or severity of ART side effects and adverse reactions (**Box 3**).[36–38]

Antiretroviral treatment and the perinatal period

HIV-positive women who are planning to become or are already pregnant should be reassured that the benefits of ART outweigh the risks in pregnancy and that optimal

---

Box 2
Antiretroviral treatment adherence barriers for human immunodeficiency virus–positive women

More severe and/or frequent side effects and adverse reactions

More barriers to obtaining ART (eg, financial, transportation)

More likely to have ART adherence challenges (eg, less control over lives, homelessness, stigma, caregiving responsibilities)

More mental health problems impeding self-care

Substance use/abuse impeding self-care, increasing risks (eg, trading sex for drugs)

More interpersonal or other violence impeding self-care

Data from Barroso J. Psychosocial issues, mental health, and substance abuse. Rockville (MD): US Department of Health and Human Services (DHHS), Health Resources and Services Administration (HRSA); 2013. p. 339.

---

reduction in maternal-to-child HIV transmission and improved maternal health depend upon initiating potent ART promptly.[23,37,38] ART side effects may mimic and exacerbate unpleasant pregnancy symptoms. Maternity care providers should educate patients to recognize and report side effects and potentially dangerous adverse reactions and to use self-care practices to reduce their impacts or occurrence.[25,38] Maternity care providers must monitor patients for adverse reactions regularly and intervene promptly when these are reported.

Because of concerns over teratogenic effects in nonhuman primates, prescription of efavirenz (EFV) has largely been restricted in women planning a future pregnancy.[36] As of October 26, 2016, because of the lack of evidence of increased neural tube defects with EFV use in pregnancy, the restriction on the use of this drug in early pregnancy was removed from the maternal ART guidelines.[37] This update emphasized that EFV-containing ART should not be stopped in women diagnosed with early pregnancy if this regimen is well tolerated and effectively controlling their disease.[37]

ART adherence can falter during the postpartum period.[25] The typical challenges of this period, such as lack of sleep, hormonal changes, feeling sad, and newborn care, added to the responsibility of administering Zidovudine to the baby for HIV prevention and the worry over whether the baby will test HIV positive can lead to women neglecting their own health.[25]

Box 3
Antiretroviral medications causing more adverse effects in women

Nevirapine, a nonnucleoside reverse transcriptase inhibitor:
  Severe liver toxicity

Zidovudine, stavudine, and didanosine, nucleoside reverse transcriptase inhibitors (NRTIs) no longer recommended in the United States but possibly still in use:
  A potentially fatal complication called lactic acidosis

Regimens containing tenofovir disoproxil fumarate, an NRTI, and/or ritonavir-boosted protease inhibitors:
  Bone loss

Data from Refs.[36–38]

Antiretroviral treatment and hormonal contraception

Hormonal contraception and ART may interact adversely. Some protease inhibitors, EFV, and the integrase inhibitor, elvitegravir/cobicistat, may decrease or increase blood levels of combined oral contraceptives (COCs), and COCs may decrease the levels of the unboosted protease inhibitor, fosamprenavir.[36,39] No form of hormonal contraception, unless clearly contraindicated, should be withheld due to these interactions, especially when the contraceptive method is strongly preferred by the woman.[36] However, measures should be taken to mitigate adverse effects of interactions, for example, latex condom use where there is potential for decreased hormonal contraceptive effectiveness or use of the lowest dose of hormone when levels of one or the other or both medications may be elevated by their concomitant use.[35,36] In addition, use of unboosted fosamprenavir should be avoided in female patients desiring COCs.[35] The latest guidance from the US Medical Eligibility Criteria for Contraceptive Use[39] should be consulted for detailed contraceptive and ART interactions and updates.

Metabolic and Cardiovascular Effects of Human Immunodeficiency Virus and Antiretroviral Treatment on Women

HIV-positive women are more susceptible to fat deposition changes, particularly in the breasts and abdomen, because of HIV disease and some antiretroviral medications.[40] These body composition changes can cause distress and may inhibit ART adherence, and they are associated with elevations in lipids and glucose.[40] Traditional cardiovascular disease (CVD) risk factors of tobacco abuse, hypertension, hyperlipidemia, diabetes, and aging together with the effects of HIV and ART have resulted in higher prevalence of CVD in those with HIV relative to the general population.[41] Heart disease is the leading cause of death among HIV-positive individuals.[41] In women, the symptoms of CVD can be atypical and left unevaluated and untreated longer because they are assumed to be at low risk.[41] Thus, care of HIV-positive women must involve risk assessment and more aggressive evaluation, treatment, and risk reduction with regard to CVD.

Disease Screening in Human Immunodeficiency Virus–Positive Women

Screening recommendations for HIV-positive women can mirror those of the general population but should take into account life expectancy, individualized risk assessment, and harms and benefits of the screening.[42] For women who have a life expectancy of at least 5 to 10 years, most screening recommendations should reflect those for the general population (US Preventive Services Task Force [USPSTF]).[42,43] For women with limited life expectancy, it is essential to assess the harms versus the benefits of any screening test and ensure that the latter outweighs the former.[42]

Cancer screening

Although use of ART has led to decreases in AIDS-defining cancers like cervical cancer, the increased prevalence of HIV in older individuals and the fact that people live longer with HIV, have other conditions like hepatitis, and/or continue risky habits have contributed to greater incidences of non-AIDS–defining cancers like hepatocellular carcinoma (HCC), lung cancer, and anal cancer.[42] HIV-positive women who have a good prognosis and no high-risk genetic markers should follow the USPSTF guidelines with regard to breast, colon, and lung cancer screening.[42,43] The USPSTF currently makes no recommendations for screening for HCC or anal cancer for any population.[43]

Anogenital cancer screening in women with human immunodeficiency virus
HIV-positive women have higher rates of human papilloma virus (HPV) infection, including high-risk types, and more persistent HPV infection than uninfected women.[44] Experts recommend that HIV-positive women get cervical Pap test screening more frequently than uninfected women, that is, upon entry into HIV care, 6 months later, and then annually without high-risk HPV cotesting.[40,44] Any visible genital lesion or a Pap test showing atypical squamous cells of undetermined significance or worse should prompt a colposcopic examination with biopsy.[44]

Regular cervical Pap test screening and prompt treatment of precancerous lesions have reduced the risk for invasive cervical cancer (ICC) in HIV-positive women to that of uninfected women.[44] Still, women living with HIV who are not screened regularly have greater risks for ICC at a younger age, more advanced disease and atypical metastases, and poorer outcomes than uninfected women with a similar stage of ICC.[44] Providing HPV vaccination to HIV-positive adolescents and young adults is a practice that may reduce incidence of precancerous lesions and ICC in HIV-positive women.[44]

Anal Pap tests and digital rectal examinations may be performed on the same schedule recommended above for cervical Pap tests, but this practice is not standard because of insufficient data on harms versus benefits.[40] Women with abnormal cervical Pap tests and/or visible anogenital warts might benefit from this screening.[40] What is crucial in deciding to do anal Pap tests is ensuring that there are accessible specialists who can evaluate abnormal findings and treat precancerous lesions.

Other disease screenings
The USPSTF screening guidelines can be consulted for the timing of several other screenings.[43] Recommended frequencies of some screenings are more aggressive and specific for HIV-positive women. Depression, domestic or other violence, and alcohol, drug, and tobacco use screening should occur at the initial visit, annually, and when clinically indicated in HIV-positive women.[40] Although bone density testing is recommended at age 65 for all women, women with HIV may benefit from this testing as early as age 50 due to having more risks for premature bone loss, such as HIV disease itself, use of certain types of ART, earlier menopause, premenopausal amenorrhea, alcohol abuse, smoking, and vitamin D deficiency.[40,44] The importance of assessing HIV-positive women for CVD risk factors was discussed earlier, and this should include checking blood pressure, glucose, and lipids.

Viral hepatitis screening is recommended upon entry into care and as clinically indicated, but screening for other infectious diseases, including syphilis, gonorrhea, Chlamydia, and trichomoniasis, visually inspecting the vulva, vagina, and cervix, and performing a pelvic examination are recommended upon entry into care, as clinically indicated, and annually for sexually active HIV-positive women.[40,44] These latter assessments are important not just for public health but also for the health of individual women because STDs can worsen HIV disease (in the case of herpes simplex virus type 2) and increase risks for HIV reinfection and maternal-to-child HIV transmission and incidence of pelvic inflammatory disease.[44]

General Psychosocial Needs and Care of Human Immunodeficiency Virus–Positive Women

More so than men, women living with HIV may need transportation, housing, childcare, and food assistance and help applying for health coverage and navigating the health care system.[23,26] Assessment of women's current social support and spiritual practices and beliefs is important to planning care.[17,39,45] They may need peer and other formal social support or benefit from a referral to a spiritual leader or community, especially if they struggle with disclosure and are isolated.[26,45] Two intervention programs that have shown some promise in addressing psychosocial needs of HIV-positive women are described in **Box 4**.[24,46]

Other psychosocial needs include sensitively conducted and repeated assessments for violence as well as for mental health problems and substance abuse.[26] It is crucial to have professionals integrated into the primary care setting who can address and obtain urgent referrals for these problems.

Self-care practices important for women to live well with human immunodeficiency virus/AIDS

Because HIV infection has largely become a chronic disease, patient self-management is essential. Entering and remaining in care and adhering to ART are fundamental to achieving optimal health.[23] Understanding HIV disease, its treatment, and risk reduction is important to the process of engaging in care and taking on health promotion and disease prevention practices.[23] Because gaining knowledge is rarely sufficient for commitment to health behavior changes, motivation must be tapped and mobilized to aid women in setting and achieving personal health goals.[23]

To cope with the HIV stigma and make difficult decisions, women need to be open to working with behavioral health specialists, peer counselors, and others to fortify their psychological health and address harmful situations like IPV, substance abuse, and isolation.[23,26] In addition, they need to learn effective stress reduction techniques and to value and address their own needs as much as those of others.[23] In developing these techniques, prioritizing self-care, and taking some control over their health, HIV-positive women can succeed in improving self-esteem and self-efficacy and become increasingly active participants in their health care.

Abstaining from risky behaviors such as tobacco, alcohol, and illicit substance use and unprotected sex are other beneficial self-care practices for HIV-positive women.[23] If complete abstinence is not possible, women should at least reduce the risks of

---

Box 4
Interventions addressing psychosocial and other care needs of human immunodeficiency virus–positive women

The Guide to Healing Project:

Implemented with HIV-positive women of color in North Carolina:
    Strove to get women into care early
    Provided strengths-based counseling
    Taught coping, health literacy, and life skills
    Offered both informational and social support

The Women Involved in Life Learning from Other Women program (WiLLOW):

Implemented with predominantly black HIV-positive women in Alabama and Georgia

Involved four 4-hour interactive group sessions led by a female HIV educator and HIV-positive peer educator:
    Aimed to increase knowledge, change attitudes, increase self-efficacy, and teach safer sex negotiation

Data from Messer LC, Quinlivan EB, Parnell H, et al. Barriers and facilitators to testing, treatment entry, and engagement in care by HIV-positive women of color. AIDS Patient Care STDS 2013;27(7):398–407; and Wingood GM, DiClemente RJ, Mikhail I, et al. A randomized controlled trial to reduce HIV transmission risk behaviors and STDs among women living with HIV: the WiLLOW program. J Acquir Immune Defic Syndr 2004;37(Suppl 2):S58–67.

unhealthy activities such as by not sharing equipment for drug use, reducing number of sexual partners, and using condoms with most partners.[26,38,47] Engaging in health-promoting practices like getting adequate sleep, doing aerobic and weight-bearing exercise, and eating a healthy diet support wellness.[23] Diets should be sufficient in calories; low in cholesterol, saturated fats, and simple sugars; and rich in vitamins, minerals, lean protein, and fiber.[48] Finally, women should learn and follow safe food handling and preparation practices.[38,48]

SUMMARY

Although HIV-positive women in the United States face several barriers to optimal health and well-being, having access to affordable, high-quality, comprehensive, and culturally appropriate care can greatly support them in overcoming challenges and drawing upon strengths to achieve good outcomes. Health care and other service providers and patients and families must not only respect and trust one another but also be knowledgeable about HIV, ART, and best practices to promote health and prevent disease and disability in the context of HIV. Medical goals of viral suppression, immune function preservation, and avoidance of HIV/AIDS–related conditions will not be met without much attention to and assistance with psychosocial needs, at both the individual and the societal advocacy levels. Genuinely partnering with women and gaining their confidence are the first and most important steps in successfully implementing best practices and motivating women to adopt healthy behaviors and take responsibility for self-care.

REFERENCES

1. Aziz M, Smith KY. Challenges and successes in linking HIV-infected women to care in the United States. Clin Infect Dis 2011;52(Supp 2):S231–7.
2. Centers for Disease Control and Prevention (CDC). HIV among women 2017. Available at: https://www.cdc.gov/hiv/group/gender/women/index.html. Accessed June 12, 2017.
3. The Henry J. Kaiser Family Foundation. A report on women and HIV/AIDS in the United States 2013. Available at: http://www.womenhiv.org/wp-content/uploads/2013/06/KFF-2013-report-on-women-and-HIV.pdf. Accessed June 12, 2017.
4. Centers for Disease Control and Prevention (CDC). HIV in the United States: at a glance 2017. Available at: https://www.cdc.gov/hiv/statistics/overview/ataglance.html. Accessed June 5, 2017.
5. Centers for Disease Control and Prevention (CDC). HIV Surveillance Report, 2015. Available at: http://www.cdc.gov/hiv/library/reports/hiv-surveillance.html. Accessed June 5, 2017.
6. Centers for Disease Control and Prevention (CDC). Today's HIV/AIDS epidemic 2016. Available at: https://www.cdc.gov/nchhstp/newsroom/docs/factsheets/todaysepidemic-508.pdf. Accessed June 12, 2017.
7. The American Foundation for AIDS Research (amfAR). Statistics: women and HIV 2017. Available at: http://www.amfar.org/about-hiv-and-aids/facts-and-stats/statistics–women-and-hiv-aids/. Accessed June 12, 2017.
8. Centers for Disease Control and Prevention (CDC). HIV among Hispanics/Latinos 2017. Available at: https://www.cdc.gov/hiv/group/racialethnic/hispaniclatinos/index.html. Accessed June 12, 2017.
9. Centers for Disease Control and Prevention (CDC). HIV among African Americans 2017. Available at: https://www.cdc.gov/hiv/group/racialethnic/africanamericans/index.html. Accessed June 25, 2017.

10. U.S. Census Bureau. QuickFacts, people, race and Hispanic origin 2015. Available at: https://www.census.gov/quickfacts/. Accessed June 22, 2017.

11. Centers for Disease Control and Prevention (CDC). HIV in the United States: the stages of care 2012. Available at: https://www.cdc.gov/hiv/pdf/research_mmp_stagesofcare.pdf. Accessed June 10, 2017.

12. Sullivan KA, Messer LC, Quinlivan EB. Substance abuse, violence, and HIV/AIDS (SAVA) syndemic effects on viral suppression among HIV positive women of color. AIDS Patient Care STDS 2015;29(Supp 1):S42–8.

13. U.S. Department of Health and Human Services (DHHS). National HIV/AIDS Strategy for the United States: overview, 2015. Available at: https://www.hiv.gov/federal-response/national-hiv-aids-strategy/overview. Accessed June 19, 2017.

14. Greenblatt RM. Epidemiology and natural history of HIV infection in women. Rockville (MD): U.S. Department of Health and Human Services (DHHS), Health Resources and Services Administration (HRSA); 2013. p. 1–18.

15. Centers for Disease Control and Prevention (CDC). Leading causes of death in females 2014. Available at: https://www.cdc.gov/women/lcod/2014/black/index.htm. Accessed June 19, 2017.

16. U.S. Department of Health and Human Services. Health Resources and Services Administration. A guide to the clinical care of women with HIV. Rockville (MD): U.S. DHHS; 2013.

17. Dalmida SG. Spirituality, mental health, physical health, and health-related quality of life among women with HIV/AIDS: integrating spirituality into mental health care. Issues Ment Health Nurs 2014;27(2):185–98.

18. Merenstein D, Schneider MF, Cox C, et al. Association of childcare burden and household composition with adherence to HAART in the Women's Interagency Study. AIDS Patient Care STDS 2009;23(4):289–96.

19. Squires KE, Hodder SL, Feinberg J, et al. Health needs of HIV-infected women in the U.S.: insights from the women living positive survey. AIDS Patient Care STDS 2011;25(5):279–85.

20. Taylor B. HIV, stigma and health: integration of theoretical concepts and the lived experiences of individuals. J Adv Nurs 2001;35(5):792–8.

21. Centers for Disease Control and Prevention (CDC). HIV in the United States by geographic distribution 2017. Available at: https://www.cdc.gov/hiv/statistics/overview/geographicdistribution.html. Accessed June 22, 2017.

22. Breskin A, Adimora AA, Westreich D. Women and HIV in the United States. PLoS One 2017;12(2):e0172367. Available at: http://journals.plos.org/plosone/article?id=10.1371/journal.pone.0172367. Accessed June 21, 2017.

23. Anderson JR. Approach to the patient. Rockville (MD): U.S. Department of Health and Human Services (DHHS), Health Resources and Services Administration (HRSA); 2013. p. 19–36.

24. Messer LC, Quinlivan EB, Parnell H, et al. Barriers and facilitators to testing, treatment entry, and engagement in care by HIV-positive women of color. AIDS Patient Care STDS 2013;27(7):398–407.

25. Armas-Kolostroubis L, Cheever L. Adherance to HIV treatment and retention in care. Rockville (MD): U.S. Department of Health and Human Services (DHHS), Health Resources and Services Administration (HRSA); 2013. p. 133–50.

26. Barroso J. Psychosocial issues, mental health, and substance abuse. Rockville (MD): U.S. Department of Health and Human Services (DHHS), Health Resources and Services Administration (HRSA); 2013. p. 339–76.

27. Maman S, Campbell J, Sweat MD, et al. The intersections of HIV and violence: directions for future research and interventions. Soc Sci Med 2000;50(4):459–78.
28. Cook JA, Cohen MH, Burke J, et al. Effects of depressive symptoms and mental health quality of life on use of highly active antiretroviral therapy among HIV-seropositive women. J Acquir Immune Defic Syndr 2002;30:401–9.
29. Dale S, Cohen M, Weber K, et al. Abuse and resilience in relation to HAART medication adherence and HIV viral load among women with HIV in the United States. AIDS Patient Care STDS 2014;28(3):136–43.
30. Gielen AC, Ghandour RM, Burke JG, et al. HIV/AIDS and intimate partner violence: intersecting women's health issues in the United States. Trauma Violence Abuse 2007;18(2):178–98.
31. Machtinger EL, Wilson TC, Haberer JE, et al. Psychological trauma and PTSD in HIV-positive women: a meta-analysis. AIDS Behav 2012;16:2091–100.
32. Machtinger EL, Haberer JE, Wilson TC, et al. Recent trauma is associated with antiretroviral failure and HIV transmission risk behavior among HIV-positive women and female-identified transgenders. AIDS Behav 2012;16:2160–70.
33. Gielen AC, McDonnell KA, Burke JG, et al. Women's lives after an HIV-positive diagnosis: disclosure and violence. Matern Child Health J 2000;4(2):111–20.
34. Koenig LJ, Moore J. Women, violence, and HIV: a critical evaluation with implications for HIV services. Matern Child Health J 2000;4(2):103–9.
35. Aaron E, Anderson JR. Preconception care and contraception. Rockville (MD): U.S. Department of Health and Human Services (DHHS), Health Resources and Services Administration (HRSA); 2013. p. 227–61.
36. U.S. DHHS Panel on Antiretroviral Guidelines for Adults and Adolescents. Guidelines for the use of antiretroviral agents in HIV-1-infected adults and adolescents 2017. Available at: https://aidsinfo.nih.gov/guidelines/html/1/adult-and-adolescent-arv-guidelines/23/hiv-infected-women. Accessed May 21, 2017.
37. U.S. DHHS Panel on Antiretroviral Guidelines for Adults and Adolescents. Recommendations for use of antiretroviral drugs in pregnant HIV-1-infected women for maternal health and interventions to reduce perinatal HIV transmission in the United States 2017. Available at: https://aidsinfo.nih.gov/guidelines/html/3/perinatal-guidelines/0/. Accessed June 24, 2017.
38. Anderson J. HIV and pregnancy. Rockville (MD): U.S. Department of Health and Human Services (DHHS), Health Resources and Services Administration (HRSA); 2013. p. 263–338.
39. Curtis KM, Tepper NK, Jatlaoui TC, et al. U.S. medical eligibility criteria for contraceptive use. MMWR Recomm Rep 2016;65(3):1–103.
40. Feinberg J. Primary medical care. Rockville (MD): U.S. Department of Health and Human Services (DHHS), Health Resources and Services Administration (HRSA); 2013. p. 73–132.
41. Volpe M, Uglietti A, Castagna A, et al. Cardiovascular disease in women with HIV-1 infection. Int J Cardiol 2017;241:50–6.
42. Sigel K, Dubrow R, Silverberg M, et al. Cancer screening in patients infected with HIV. Curr HIV/AIDS Rep 2011;8(3):142–52.
43. U.S. Preventive Screening Task Force. Published recommendations 2017. Available at: https://www.uspreventiveservicestaskforce.org/BrowseRec/Index/browse-recommendations. Accessed June 25, 2017.
44. Anderson J. Gynecologic problems. Rockville (MD): U.S. Department of Health and Human Services (DHHS), Health Resources and Services Administration (HRSA); 2013. p. 151–226.

45. McCormick DP, Holder B, Wetsel MA, et al. Spirituality and HIV disease: an integrated perspective. J Assoc Nurses AIDS Care 2001;12(3):58–65.
46. Wingood GM, DiClemente RJ, Mikhail I, et al. A randomized controlled trial to reduce HIV transmission risk behaviors and STDs among women living with HIV: the WiLLOW program. J Acquir Immune Defic Syndr 2004;37(Supp 2): S58–67.
47. Baeten JM, Celum C. Prevention of HIV infection. Rockville (MD): U.S. Department of Health and Human Services (DHHS), Health Resources and Services Administration (HRSA); 2013. p. 39–72.
48. Academy of Nutrition and Dietetics. Nutrition tips to keep the immune system strong for people with HIV-AIDS 2016. Available at: http://www.eatright.org/resource/health/diseases-and-conditions/hiv-aids/nutrition-and-hiv-aids. Accessed June 28, 2017.

Management of Coinfections in Patients with Human Immunodeficiency Virus

Sabra S. Custer, DNP, MS, FNP-BC

KEYWORDS

- HBV • HCV • Tuberculosis • Coinfections

KEY POINTS

- Tuberculosis, hepatitis B, and hepatitis C are significant coinfections that are diagnosed in many patients with human immunodeficiency virus (HIV) and that require treatment along with HIV.
- Screening of patients with HIV for these coinfections is important to avoid progression and organ damage from the coinfection.
- Coinfected patients may require additional monitoring during treatment of the coinfection.
- Drug-drug interactions with the patient's antiretroviral regimen must be considered when treating a coinfection.

INTRODUCTION

In the age of effective antiretroviral therapy (ART), the focus and ultimate measure of healthy living with human immunodeficiency virus (HIV) infection is adherence to an effective antiretroviral (ARV) regimen and long-term virologic suppression. However, for many patients, there may be other infections that require treatment. Tuberculosis (TB), hepatitis B, and hepatitis C are significant coinfections that are diagnosed in many patients with HIV. These coinfections often remain subclinical for long periods of time but can be spread to other individuals. In addition, these coinfections can cause organ damage and systemic disease quicker in an HIV-positive patient. Therefore, it is important that clinicians working with patients with HIV appropriately screen for TB, hepatitis B, and hepatitis C and work with their patients for effective treatment when diagnosed. All 3 coinfections can be successfully treated alongside HIV infection with appropriate medication choices, monitoring for adverse effects, and ongoing patient education.

Disclosure: The author has no financial relationships to disclose.
College of Nursing, University of South Carolina, 1601 Greene Street, Columbia, SC 29208, USA
E-mail address: Sabra.custer@sc.edu

Nurs Clin N Am 53 (2018) 83–96
https://doi.org/10.1016/j.cnur.2017.10.001
0029-6465/18/© 2017 Elsevier Inc. All rights reserved.

TUBERCULOSIS STATISTICS

Worldwide prevalence of TB is hard to determine accurately, but the Centers for Disease Control and Prevention (CDC) estimates that approximately one-third of the global population is infected.[1] The World Health Organization (WHO) estimates that 10.4 million new cases occurred worldwide in 2015, including 1.2 million cases of coinfections with HIV.[2] In 2015, there were an estimated 1.4 million deaths caused by TB, and another 400,000 TB-related deaths in persons coinfected with HIV and TB.[2] From 2000 to 2015 there were slight reductions in the worldwide number of deaths caused by TB; the incidence declined slightly (by 1.5%) from 2014 to 2015.[2] However, TB remained in the top 10 causes of death in 2015, outranking HIV.[1] Approximately 11% of persons diagnosed with TB in 2015 were also HIV positive, with the highest proportion of diagnosed coinfections occurring in Africa and southern Africa. Approximately 5% of worldwide TB cases diagnosed in 2015 were determined to be drug resistant.[2]

Although the United States is not a high-burden country per WHO guidelines, TB is still a significant concern there. The CDC reported 9287 new cases in 2016, which translates to a rate of 2.9 cases per 100,000 people. Although the absolute incidence in 2015 increased from previous years, overall population increase has resulted in a generally stable incidence rate over the last 4 years.[3] The last nationwide TB prevalence estimate was obtained via the 2011 to 2012 National Health and Nutrition Examination Survey (NHANES). Through laboratory testing, approximately 5% of this nationwide sample was determined to be positive for TB.[4] Data on drug-resistant TB in the United States are only available for 2015; approximately 1% of cases diagnosed that year were drug resistant.[3]

In addition to considering HIV-positive individuals as a subset of all persons infected with TB, clinicians working with HIV-positive patients should be aware that a significant percentage of the HIV-positive population may be also be infected with TB. In 2015, in 12 WHO high-burden countries, 10% of persons newly enrolled in HIV care were also diagnosed with TB that same year, indicating the significance of TB as an opportunistic infection or coinfection.[2] In the United States, the percentage of persons who are diagnosed annually with both TB and HIV has significantly decreased, from 48.2% in 1993 to 5.5% in 2015.[5] This improvement was likely caused by advances in HIV treatment, but a 5.5% coinfection rate still represents a significant portion of the HIV-positive population.

TUBERCULOSIS SCREENING

The high rate of coinfection with TB in HIV-positive individuals and the increasing risk of progression to active disease highlight the need for appropriate screening in clients who are HIV positive. Current treatment guidelines recommend TB screening at the time of HIV diagnosis regardless of risk factors for TB exposure.[6] Because significant immunosuppression, generally considered a CD4 count less than 200 cells/μL, can cause a false-negative result, retesting is recommended once the individual's CD4 count improves even if the initial TB screening was negative.[6] Continuing with annual TB screening is only recommended if the person has ongoing likely exposure to TB.[6]

Historically, screening for latent TB infection (LTBI) was performed with a tuberculin skin test (TST), which is an intradermal injection of *Mycobacterium tuberculosis* antigens and depends on a cell-mediated immune response to indicate infection with *M tuberculosis*.[7] Drawbacks of the TST include the possibility of mistakes in performing an intradermal injection, the need to return to a health care provider to have the test interpreted, the inherent subjectivity of measuring the induration, and the possibility of false-positive results in certain individuals, such as those with previous bacillus Calmette-Guérin (BCG) vaccination or infection with non-TB mycobacteria.[8] In the general population, an induration of greater than or equal to 15 mm is considered positive for TB infection but, in the HIV-positive population, an induration of greater than or equal to 5 mm is considered positive.[9]

Beginning in 2001, the US Food and Drug Administration (FDA) began approving new blood-based tests called interferon-gamma release assays (IGRAs), which still test cell-mediated immune response to specific *M tuberculosis* antigens but offer several advantages compared with the TST. IGRAs do not require a return visit, provide a quantitative result based on machine measurement of enzyme reactions in a blood sample, and are less prone to false-positive results caused by BCG vaccination or infection with other mycobacteria species.[7] In most cases, current screening guidelines recommend the use of IGRA tests, especially if the person being tested is unlikely to return for the TST reading.[8]

At present, there are 2 IGRAs approved by the FDA for TB screening: the Quanti-FERON TB Gold In Tube (QFT-GIT) and the T-SPOT.TB test (T-SPOT).[10] Both are quantitative tests based on enzyme-linked assays, but the QFT-GIT directly measures interferon-gamma concentration in the plasma, whereas the T-SPOT counts T cells that are releasing interferon-gamma.[8] Although the early IGRA tests required a tight timeline to transport blood samples to the laboratory for processing, recent improvements have extended the minimum interval between obtaining the sample and conducting the assay such that this is no longer a significant barrier in most settings.[7]

Because of slightly different numerical cutoffs for IGRA tests and other differences in methodology, there is variation in published sensitivity and specificity for these tests. Sensitivities for the QFT-GIT and T-SPOT have ranged from a low of 70% in some studies to 94% in others.[7] In general, the QFT-GIT and T-SPOT tests are considered to have equal sensitivity to the TST. IGRAs should be more specific than the TST because of the use of specific antigens and lack of false-positive results in individuals with BCG vaccination. Published studies have found QFT-GIT specificity at 99%.[7] More and larger studies are needed to validate the specificity of the T-SPOT.[7] Studies regarding possible differences in accuracy of IGRA assays specifically among immunocompromised patients are limited and have conflicting results. The most important variable in patients who are HIV positive and being screened for TB is the CD4 count. Lower CD4 count increases the risk for false-negative results on all 3 tests for LTBI.[7]

DIAGNOSIS OF TUBERCULOSIS DISEASE

An important aspect of clinical treatment is the understanding of the difference between LTBI and active TB, or TB disease. Screening tests such as the TST or IGRAs, previously discussed, simply indicate an immune system response to the *M tuberculosis* antigen. Additional testing is necessary to further determine whether the individual has only LTBI or active TB disease. Persons with only LTBI are not infectious to others and should have no physical symptoms or respiratory problems. However, persons with TB disease usually show evidence of lung tissue damage on a chest radiograph, report systemic symptoms, and are infectious to those around them.[9] Estimates of the likelihood of LTBI converting to TB disease vary; however, immunosuppression is a known risk factor that increases the risk of developing TB disease. For individuals who are HIV positive, the lifetime risk of LTBI converting to TB disease is approximately 20%, which is higher than in the general population.[11]

On diagnosis of LTBI, the clinician must then screen the patient for TB disease. Diagnosis of TB disease includes screening for common symptoms, imaging of the lungs, and laboratory testing of sputum samples.[8,12] Thorough questioning regarding symptoms of TB is essential. Constitutional symptoms include weight loss, fatigue, night sweats, anorexia, and fever. Symptoms of pulmonary disease include chronic cough, hemoptysis, and chest pain.[13] HIV-positive individuals may have markedly different symptoms, such as extrapulmonary infection sites and nontraditional symptoms, especially if their CD4 counts are less than 200 cells/μL. Significant immunosuppression from HIV infection may result in more severe systemic TB symptoms but also reduce the likelihood of classic chest radiograph changes, even in pulmonary TB disease.[13] The presence of TB-suggestive symptoms should prompt imaging of the chest, most commonly a chest radiograph. Evidence of disease activity in the lungs should then be followed with sputum sampling.[8,10]

A microscopic examination of a sputum smear for the presence of acid-fast bacilli (AFB) is the primary microbiological test for TB disease with pulmonary involvement.[8] The sensitivity of a single sputum smear is only estimated at 54%, but the overall sensitivity increases to around 70% with the testing of 3 sequential morning samples.[8] There is no significant difference in sensitivity of sputum smears between immunocompetent and immunocompromised patients.[10] Samples that are positive for AFB should also be cultured for M tuberculosis growth, but this takes up to 4 weeks depending on the culture method.[8] As an adjunct test to both AFB smear microscopy and culture, nucleic acid amplification testing (NAAT) is recommended in the most recent screening guidelines.[8] NAAT can detect the specific M tuberculosis species and provides results much more quickly than either liquid or solid culture medium. The sensitivity and specificity of NAAT varies with the AFB smear results and overall suspicion of disease.[8] Rapid molecular tests for isoniazid (INH) and rifampin resistance are available and are highly recommended in patients with HIV infection.[8,12]

TREATMENT OF LATENT TUBERCULOSIS INFECTION

For the general population, there are 3 basic options for LTBI treatment: 9 months of daily INH, 6 months of daily INH, or 3 months of weekly INH and rifapentine.[9] For HIV-positive individuals, the preferred regimen is 9 months of INH either daily or twice weekly, but 9 months of therapy is often a barrier to successful completion and there are several alternatives.[14] Rifampin or rifabutin may be used exclusively for only 4 months in patients who cannot tolerate INH or have INH resistance, but they have some drug-drug interactions with ARVs, especially protease inhibitors. Several rifampin interactions can be managed with dose adjustments, but rifampin is not recommended to be coadministered with protease inhibitors.[6] The 3-month regimen of weekly INH and rifapentine can be used in HIV-positive patients as long as protease inhibitors are not part of the ARV regimen.[14] All INH-containing regimens should also include pyridoxine for prevention of peripheral neuropathy.[14] Clinicians should frequently consult the Department of Health and Human Services annual guidelines on HIV treatment for further details on drug-drug interactions between TB medications and ARVs.[6]

The need for LTBI treatment should not delay initiation of ART in patients who are also newly diagnosed with HIV infection. Immune system reconstitution also helps prevent progression of LTBI to TB disease, therefore LTBI medications and an appropriate ARV regimen should generally be started concurrently.[14] The most significant adverse effect that requires monitoring while on any regimen for LTBI is drug-induced hepatitis. Clinicians should counsel patients regarding other risk factors for hepatitis and screen for or prevent those if possible. Treatment guidelines recommend monthly monitoring visits at which patients can be asked about any symptoms of hepatitis and liver enzymes can be drawn. Increases in liver enzyme levels to 3 times the upper limit of normal generally warrant cessation of LTBI treatment.[14]

TREATMENT OF TUBERCULOSIS DISEASE

Treatment of active TB, or TB disease, requires multiple medications and is inherently more complicated than treatment of LTBI, both in monoinfected patients and in those coinfected with HIV. For most patients with HIV, if they are concurrently diagnosed with both HIV and TB disease, TB medications should be started immediately and ART should be started within 2 to 8 weeks. Patients with HIV who have CD4 counts less than 200 cells/μL and/or have HIV-related complications at the time of diagnosis need ART initiation sooner.[12]

General principles of TB disease treatment include a 2-month induction phase with 3 or 4 active drugs followed by a 4-month to 7-month continuation phase of 2 drugs, initiation of empiric treatment in cases that are highly suspicious while awaiting confirmation of TB disease, and the use of directly observed therapy (DOT) to improve adherence and outcomes in certain patient populations.[15] As part of the diagnosis process, the sputum samples should be tested for sensitivity to the first-line drugs so that this information is available during the planning of treatment. For the general population, DOT may be used at a frequency of only 3 days a week, but 7 or 5 days a week is preferable, especially in patients coinfected with HIV.[12,14] **Table 1**, from the CDC, provides an overview of the 4 most common regimens for TB disease that is susceptible to all first-line drugs.[16] Not reflected in **Table 1** is the recommendation that ethambutol is unnecessary during the intensive phase if the M tuberculosis strain is susceptible to INH, rifampin, and pyrazinamide.[14]

Monitoring during treatment of TB disease should include monthly sputum samples until 2 consecutive samples are negative; a repeat chest radiograph 2 months into treatment if the initial sputum sample was negative, as a way to monitor for improvement of pulmonary appearance; and laboratory testing for liver enzymes. Patients should also be interviewed frequently regarding symptomatic improvement, any adverse effects of medications, and their adherence to the TB medications.[14] Patients who are coinfected with HIV and on ARVs are at higher risk of drug-induced hepatitis caused by drug-drug interactions. Coinfected patients with very low initial CD4 counts who start ARVs early are at higher risk of TB immune reconstitution inflammatory syndrome (IRIS), which is likely to entail worsening of pulmonary or systemic TB symptoms. IRIS may be treated with nonsteroidal or steroidal antiinflammatory drugs while both TB medications and ARVs are continued.[12]

HEPATITIS B STATISTICS

Worldwide, hepatitis B virus (HBV) is the most common cause of liver disease.[14] Because of the similar modes of transmission and efficiency of infection, approximately 10% of HIV-positive individuals are coinfected with hepatitis B.[14] Although approximately 6% to 10% of monoinfected adults remain chronically infected following contraction of the virus, this percentage is higher in coinfected patients at around 10% to 15%.[12,17] In addition, in coinfected patients whose hepatitis B infection remains chronic, it is more likely that HBV viral levels will remain higher and therefore be more likely to cause liver disease and possible liver cancer.[12] Therefore it is vital that newly diagnosed patients with HIV be screened for HBV. Patients who are negative for hepatitis B infection should be vaccinated with the 3-dose series or with the combination hepatitis A and hepatitis B vaccine if they need protection from both viruses.[14]

Table 1
Drug-susceptible tuberculosis disease treatment regimens

Regimen	Intensive Phase Drugs[a]	Intensive Phase Interval and Dose[b] (Minimum Duration)	Continuation Phase Drugs	Continuation Phase Interval and Dose[b,c] (Minimum Duration)	Range of Total Doses	Comments[c,d]
1	INH RIF PZA EMB	7 d/wk for 56 doses (8 wk) or 5 d/wk for 40 doses (8 wk)	INH RIF	7 d/wk for 126 doses (18 wk) or 5 d/wk for 90 doses (18 wk)	182–130	This is the preferred regimen for patients with newly diagnosed pulmonary TB
2	INH RIF PZA EMB	7 d/wk for 56 doses (8 wk) or 5 d/wk for 40 doses (8 wk)	INH RIF	3 times weekly for 54 doses (18 wk)	110–94	Preferred alternative regimen in situations in which more frequent DOT during continuation phase is difficult to achieve
3	INH RIF PZA EMB	3 times weekly for 24 doses (8 wk)	INH RIF	3 times weekly for 54 doses (18 wk)	78	Use regimen with caution in patients with HIV and/or cavitary disease. Missed doses can lead to treatment failure, relapse, and acquired drug resistance
4	INH RIF PZA EMB	7 d/wk for 14 doses then twice weekly for 12 doses[e]	INH RIF	Twice weekly for 36 doses (18 wk)	62	Do not use twice-weekly regimens in patients infected with HIV or patients with smear-positive and/or cavitary disease. If doses are missed then therapy is equivalent to once weekly, which is inferior

Regimen Effectiveness: Greater → Lesser

Note: Use of once-weekly therapy with INH 900 mg and rifapentine 600 mg in the continuation phase is not generally recommended. In uncommon situations in which more than once-weekly DOT is difficult to achieve, once-weekly continuation-phase therapy with INH 900 mg plus rifapentine 600 mg may be considered for use only in patients not infected with HIV without cavitation on chest radiography.

Abbreviations: EMB, ethambutol; PZA, pyrazinamide; RIF, rifampin.

[a] Other combinations may be appropriate in certain circumstances; additional details are provided by Nahid and colleagues.[15]

[b] When DOT is used, drugs may be given 5 d/wk and the necessary number of doses adjusted accordingly. Although there are no studies that compare 5 with 7 daily doses, extensive experience indicates this would be an effective practice. DOT should be used when drugs are administered less than 7 d/wk.

[c] Based on expert opinion, patients with cavitation on initial chest radiograph and positive cultures at completion of 2 months of therapy should receive a 7-month (31-week) continuation phase.

[d] Pyridoxine (vitamin B₆), 25–50 mg/d, is given with INH to all persons at risk of neuropathy (eg, pregnant women; breastfeeding infants; persons with HIV; patients with diabetes, alcoholism, malnutrition, or chronic renal failure; or patients with advanced age). For patients with peripheral neuropathy, experts recommend increasing pyridoxine dose to 100 mg/d.

[e] Alternatively, some US TB control programs have administered intensive-phase regimens 5 d/wk for 15 doses (3 weeks), then twice weekly for 12 doses.

From Nahid P, Dorman SE, Alipanah N, et al. Official American Thoracic Society/Centers for Disease Control and Prevention/Infectious Diseases Society of America Clinical Practice Guidelines: Treatment of Drug-Susceptible Tuberculosis. Clin Infect Dis 2016;63(7):856; with permission.

HEPATITIS B SCREENING AND DIAGNOSIS

Because of the structure and genetic material of HBV, there are multiple types of antigens and antibodies that can be detected in a blood sample for screening. The hepatitis B early antigen (HbeAg) and surface antigen (HbsAg) and the early, core, and surface antibodies (anti-Hbe, anti-Hbc, and anti-Hbs respectively) are used in combination to determine the stage of infection and immunity to future infection caused by either previous infection or immunity. The CDC provides an excellent reference document on hepatitis B serologies and online training modules.[17,18] The remainder of this article focuses on diagnosis and treatment of chronic hepatitis B, because patients who remain chronically infected are at increased risk of liver disease and damage. Chronic HBV is diagnosed by the presence of HbsAg, HbeAg, or the presence of HBV DNA twice over a period of at least 6 months. Patients with chronic HBV are also likely to have total anti-Hbc (immunoglobulin [Ig] M and IgG).[18]

Once chronic HBV is diagnosed, further testing is necessary for information regarding liver function. Patients should have a complete blood count and their liver enzymes, albumin, bilirubin, and prothrombin levels should be checked at the time of diagnosis and every 6 months thereafter to monitor liver inflammation and function. Assessment for fibrotic changes in the liver can be done by various methods, including noninvasive testing by transient elastography. In those with evidence of cirrhosis or with other risk factors for liver cancer (eg, Asian ethnicity, increasing age, adult men from sub-Saharan Africa) should also undergo liver ultrasonography every 6 months to screen for liver cancer.[14] Other predicted care includes vaccination against hepatitis A if necessary, counseling to avoid alcohol or other hepatotoxic substances and medications, and screening for hepatitis C.[12,14] Because of the likelihood of higher levels of HBV DNA in coinfected individuals, it is important that they receive counseling on preventing HBV transmission to others, although prevention strategies for HBV transmission equate those for HIV transmission prevention.

HEPATITIS B TREATMENT

Because of dual activity of many HBV medications and the shared goals of viral suppression in both chronic HBV and HIV treatment, chronic HBV treatment is often subsumed within the patient's ARV regimen. Effective chronic HBV treatment can achieve the disappearance of HbsAg and long-term HBV DNA suppression, which is considered an immunologic cure.[19] Medications currently approved for treating HBV include interferon and 4 nucleotide analogue drugs. Most of the nucleotide analogue drugs also have anti-HIV activity.[19] When diagnoses of both HIV and chronic HBV are made concurrently, the patient should start treatment of both simultaneously. The ARV regimen must include 2 drugs with activity against HBV, preferably tenofovir disoproxil fumarate (TDF) and emtricitabine, at the standard dosage and frequency for HIV treatment.[19] In November 2016, a newer form of TDF, tenofovir alafenamide fumarate (TAF), was approved by the FDA for treatment of HBV as well as HIV. TAF has several benefits compared with TDF, including reduced nephrotoxicity and reduced effect on bone mineral density because of its conversion to the active form of the drug only once it reaches the intracellular space.[20,21] TAF is also available in a combination pill with emtricitabine for ease of administration.[22] Use of 2 ARVs with activity against HBV is necessary because only 1 drug in the ARV regimen with activity against HBV can result in development of drug resistance in the HBV.[14]

When the dual-purpose nucleotide analogue drugs are used in coinfected patients, treatment should continue indefinitely to maintain both HBV and HIV suppression. Patients who stop the anti-HBV drugs for any reason should have their liver enzyme levels monitored frequently for acute hepatitis and the drugs may need to be reinstituted to prevent fatal outcomes.[14] In the rare cases in which a patient coinfected with HBV/HIV refuses or for any reason does not start HIV treatment immediately but requires and agrees to HBV treatment, interferon alone is the recommended treatment.[14]

When a coinfected patient is taking tenofovir (the TDF or TAF form) and emtricitabine, there are no new adverse effects of concern to clinicians treating HIV, because these drugs are well known from their long-term use in ARV regimens. Of greatest concern with tenofovir is the potential for renal tubule damage and a modest reduction in bone mineral density.[12] Interferon has more significant and unique adverse effects, such as flulike symptoms; possible significant depression; insomnia or anxiety; or other systemic symptoms of gastrointestinal distress, joint pain, or skin reactions.[14] Patients taking interferon for HBV treatment need instruction on injection techniques and closer monitoring for adverse effects. One advantage of interferon treatment is its limited duration of 48 weeks rather than indefinite treatment with the nucleotide analogues.[14]

HEPATITIS C STATISTICS

Because of sampling procedures and the likelihood of high-risk populations being missed in national surveys, it is challenging to accurately estimate the current prevalence of persons with hepatitis C virus (HCV). A recent meta-analysis that included additional sources to account for underrepresented populations determined the current United States prevalence of HCV to be between 2.5 million and 4.7 million, or 0.8% to 1.5% of the population.[23] HCV is known to cause more deaths annually than the next 60 nationally reportable infectious diseases.[24] HCV is transmitted primarily through percutaneous exposures to blood via intravenous needles, receipt of large amounts of blood through transfusion, or perinatal infection. Infection is possible through intercourse with an infected person but this is not an efficient means of transmission.[25] Although a small percentage of infected individuals may experience some acute symptoms, HCV is generally considered a chronic infection. Approximately 20% to 30% of HIV-positive patients in the United States are coinfected with HCV, likely influenced by shared modes of transmission.[14]

HEPATITIS C SCREENING AND DIAGNOSIS

Diagnosis of HCV is made with a positive serum antibody test and confirmation of active infection with an HCV viral load. Because HCV has approximately 6 genotypes that are significant when treatment is initiated, genotype testing should be conducted as part of the overall evaluation.[26] Approximately 15% to 25% of persons clear the virus on their own for unknown reasons and therefore do not require any further treatment or monitoring. If the virus is still detectable at 6 months or longer after diagnosis, this is considered chronic infection and the person is unlikely to ever spontaneously clear the virus.[24] For most patients, who remain chronically infected, between 4% and 24% are likely to develop cirrhosis after 20 years of infection.[27] Variables associated with quicker progression to cirrhosis include older age at infection, alcohol consumption, and male sex.[28] Although HCV likely has little effect on HIV progression, HCV progresses more quickly to fibrosis or hepatocellular cancer in patients who are coinfected.[12] Progression to hepatic cancer is 5 times higher and progression to cirrhosis is 10 times higher in coinfected patients compared with monoinfected patients.[29] With these considerations in mind, HIV-positive patients who are coinfected with HCV require additional monitoring and interventions to protect the liver. They should be advised to avoid or limit alcohol use, avoid hepato-toxic drugs and excess acetaminophen, be educated on preventing HCV transmission, be vaccinated for hepatitis A and B if applicable, be screened for liver cancer every 6 to 12 months, and be evaluated for potential treatment. If discovered simultaneously, patients who are coinfected should begin ART without delay both for control of HIV and for the secondary benefit of slowing HCV hepatic damage.[12] Use of ART to control HIV can mitigate at least some of the quicker progression of HCV.[12]

HEPATITIS C TREATMENT

Until the introduction and approval of the first direct-acting antivirals (DAAs) in 2011, the primary combination for treatment of HCV was pegylated interferon and ribavirin.[30] These medications caused high rates of significant adverse effects and achieved a cure in less than 50% of patients with the most common genotype.[31] The first HCV protease inhibitor drugs, telaprevir and boceprevir, increased cure rates but still had high pill burdens and serious adverse effects and are no longer recommended treatments.[29] Another generation of DAAs was approved and became integrated into treatment regimens in 2013 and 2014. These newest HCV drugs initially had to be used in combination with pegylated interferon and/or ribavirin but in the last 2 to 3 years several have gained approval as monotherapy. Cure rates on these newest regimens are 90% and more.[30] An additional improvement in the modern treatment regimens is shortened durations; many of the current DAA-only regimens can be used for only 12 weeks and some for only 8 weeks in the absence of cirrhosis.[32]

When translating the newest HCV treatments to the HIV/HCV coinfected population, clinicians must consider the potential effects of drug-drug interactions, overlapping adverse effects, and the possible unique effects of treating HCV in immunosuppressed individuals. In general, the guidelines for treating HCV in coinfected patients include minimum length of 12 weeks for HCV treatment, continuation of ART while HCV treatment is in progress, and close monitoring for HCV medication adverse effects and drug-drug interactions.[33]

Before initiating HCV treatment, all patients need a thorough clinical evaluation. In general, this includes an assessment of liver fibrosis; confirmation of the patient's HCV genotype; recent HCV viral load; bloodwork such as serum albumin, bilirubin, and platelet count to calculate cirrhosis or decompensated liver disease; renal and liver function tests; screening for alcohol or substance abuse; and extensive counseling regarding the necessary adherence to HCV therapy for success.[14] Recent advances in noninvasive methods to determine liver fibrosis, such as elastography, have simplified this part of the pretreatment evaluation.

In addition, patients who are coinfected should have a demonstrated ability to adhere to ART. Also, clinicians must consult current detailed guidelines to determine whether any changes to the patient's ART regimen are necessary to accommodate the HCV medications.[14] If a change to the ARV regimen is necessary, this should be done a few weeks in advance of initiating HCV treatment so that an undetectable HIV viral load can be confirmed and the patient can be screened for any adverse effects from the new ARVs before HCV antivirals are added to the mix. Because every class of ARVs can have significant pharmacokinetic interactions with the newer HCV DAAs, clinicians who are going to treat HCV must consult an expert and/or current detailed guidelines to check for interactions. Two excellent sources for drug-drug interactions are the Department of Health and Human Services' Guidelines for the Use of Antiretroviral Agents in HIV-1-Infected Adults and Adolescents, updated annually, found at http://www.aidsinfo.nih.gov/ContentFiles/AdultandAdolescentGL.pdf and the American Association for the Study of Liver Diseases online HCV guidelines, available at http://www.hcvguidelines.org/.[6,34] The AASLD guidelines are updated frequently as new treatments become available.

While on treatment, patients should be evaluated regularly for impairment in renal function, further increase of liver enzyme levels, and adherence to their HCV medications (and ARVs if coinfected), and should have periodic testing of HCV viral loads to determine virologic responses. An undetectable HCV level at 4 weeks of treatment is considered a rapid virologic response, undetectable HCV level at 12 weeks is an early virologic response (EVR), and maintenance of an undetectable HCV level 24 weeks after completion of therapy is considered a sustained virologic response (SVR). SVR is used by most clinicians as a standard of cure. Patients who do not achieve EVR are unlikely to ever achieve an undetectable HCV viral load and should be carefully evaluated for the usefulness of continuing therapy.[35]

EFFECTS OF COINFECTION TREATMENT ON QUALITY OF LIFE

The clinical benefits of curing TB disease and HCV and long-term suppression of HBV are well established in both the monoinfected and coinfected populations. Elimination of active replication of M tuberculosis prevents or arrests significant lung damage, respiratory dysfunction, and possible systemic morbidities.[16] Sustained suppression of both HBV and HCV should significantly reduce the risk of liver fibrosis, cirrhosis, liver failure, and hepatocellular carcinoma.[12] Less understood or recognized are the effects of treatment on quality of life for patients who are coinfected with HIV and TB, HBV, or HCV. The improvements gained in health-related quality of life (HRQOL) after successful treatment of these coinfections can improve healthy living for HIV-positive individuals.

At diagnosis, patients with active or pulmonary TB consistently report poorer HRQOL and higher levels of depression than patients with LTBI or those negative for TB.[36–39] Physical symptoms of TB disease and social stigma, anxiety, and isolation are possible contributing factors. However, in both single studies and systematic reviews, treatment of active TB has been associated with increases in HRQOL. Bauer and colleagues[37] found in a longitudinal cohort study that although patients with active TB had lower scores on the mental component summary (MCS) of the Short Form 36 (SF-36) scale (a common assessment of HRQOL), the MCS scores steadily improved over the course of treatment up to 12 months after diagnosis. Another cohort study comparing patients with active TB or LTBI found that the initial lower scores for HRQOL and higher depression at diagnosis had improved in most domains after 6 months of treatment.[38] Another recent study also found that initially impaired quality of life scores in patients with pulmonary TB improved after treatment.[40]

One study examined the effects of TB treatment on HRQOL in HIV-positive patients, and results were similar to the previously mentioned studies: on an HIV-specific measure of HRQOL, participants on treatment of TB showed significant increases in HRQOL at each time interval from baseline to a year.[41] From this HIV-specific study and the more numerous studies conducted in monoinfected patients, clinicians treating HIV can be reasonably confident when counseling their patients regarding treatment of TB disease that treatment will improve their quality of life and boost their ability to live healthily with HIV.

In addition to the obvious clinical benefits of slowing or arresting liver damage, treatment of HBV and HCV also improves quality of life and adds to healthy living for patients coinfected with one of these infections and HIV. Negative associations have been found between HBV and HRQOL in a few studies, but these have mostly been cross-sectional studies that cannot show causality or long-term benefits of HBV suppression on quality of life.[42–44] Clinicians can still reasonably conclude that avoidance or reduction of HBV morbidities maintains or improves quality of life in HIV-positive patients, but the research evidence is weak.

HCV treatment and its effect on HRQOL has been studied more extensively, and there are some published longitudinal studies showing improvement in HRQOL during and after treatment.[45–47] In addition to showing general improvements in HRQOL at the end of or after treatment, these studies also compared the newer interferon-free regimens with older interferon-based regimens and validated that treatment with interferon-free regimens was associated with fewer adverse effects and better HRQOL outcomes. Only 1 of these studies was conducted among coinfected individuals, but the results of improved HRQOL outcomes after HCV treatment in monoinfected patients can reasonably be extended to those coinfected with HIV.[46]

SUMMARY

Because of both shared modes of transmission and the immunosuppressive effects of HIV infection, HIV-positive patients are at increased risk of TB, hepatitis B, and hepatitis C. In addition, HIV-positive patients with any of these coinfections are likely to experience quicker progression and worse outcomes, such as more severe pulmonary damage and death caused by TB disease and quicker progression to cirrhosis or hepatocellular cancer from hepatitis B and C. All 3 coinfections can be successfully treated or managed in conjunction with HIV treatment, keeping in mind the potential for drug-drug interactions with the ARV regimen. When necessary, HIV providers should collaborate with specialists in TB or viral hepatitis treatment or consult the various practice guidelines summarized in this article. There is a small but consistent body of research regarding the effects of treatment of these coinfections on quality of life. The available studies found that treatment of TB, HBV, and HCV generally improves various parameters of HRQOL, especially with the advent of interferon-free regimens for HCV. Assessment of HRQOL and mental health at diagnosis of a coinfection or before considering treatment may help inform and encourage HIV-positive patients that their quality of life is likely to be improved once a coinfection is successfully treated.

REFERENCES

1. Centers for Disease Control and Prevention. Tuberculosis data and statistics. Available at: https://www.cdc.gov/tb/statistics/default.htm. Accessed June 1, 2017.
2. World Health Organization. Global TB report 2016. Available at: http://www.who.int/tb/data/en/. Accessed June 1, 2017.
3. Schmit KM, Wansaula Z, Pratt R, et al. Tuberculosis — United States, 2016. MMWR Morb Mortal Wkly Rep 2017;66:289–94.
4. Miramontes R, Hill AN, Yelk Woodruff RS, et al. Tuberculosis infection in the United States: prevalence estimates from the National Health and Nutrition Examination Survey, 2011-2012. PLoS One 2015;10(11):e0140881.
5. Centers for Disease Control and Prevention. Reported tuberculosis in the United States, 2015. Available at: http://www.cdc.gov/tb/. Accessed June 1, 2017.
6. US Department of Health and Human Services Panel on Antiretroviral Guidelines for Adults and Adolescents. Guidelines for the use of antiretroviral agents in HIV-1-infected adults and adolescents. 2016. Available at http://www.aidsinfo.nih.gov/ContentFiles/AdultandAdolescentGL.pdf. Accessed May 30, 2017.

7. Mazurek GH, Jereb J, Vernon A, et al. Updated guidelines for using interferon gamma release assays to detect mycobacterium tuberculosis infection -- United States, 2010. MMWR Recomm Rep 2010;59(RR05):1–25.

8. Lewinsohn DM, Leonard MK, LoBue PA, et al. Official American Thoracic Society/Infectious Diseases Society of America/Centers for Disease Control and Prevention clinical practice guidelines: diagnosis of tuberculosis in adults and children. Clin Infect Dis 2017;64:e1–33.

9. US Department of Health and Human Services, Centers for Disease Control and Prevention, National Center for HIV/AIDS, Viral Hepatitis, STD, and TB Prevention, Division of Tuberculosis Elimination. Latent tuberculosis infection: A guide for primary health care providers. 2013 Available at: https://www.cdc.gov/tb/publications/ltbi/pdf/targetedltbi.pdf. Accessed June 1, 2017.

10. Centers for Disease Control and Prevention. Testing for TB infection. Available at: https://www.cdc.gov/tb/topic/testing/tbtesttypes.htm. Accessed June 5, 2017.

11. Horsburgh CR Jr. Priorities for the treatment of latent tuberculosis infection in the United States. N Engl J Med 2004;350(20):2060–7.

12. Bartlett JG, Gallant JE, Pham PA. 2012 Medical management of HIV infection. Durham (NC): Johns Hopkins School of Medicine, Knowledge Source Solution; 2012.

13. Centers for Disease Control and Prevention. Diagnosing latent TB infection and TB disease. Available at: https://www.cdc.gov/tb/topic/testing/diagnosingltbi.htm. Accessed June 3, 2017.

14. US Department of Health and Human Services Panel on Opportunistic Infections in HIV-Infected Adults and Adolescents. Guidelines for the prevention and treatment of opportunistic infections in HIV-infected adults and adolescents: recommendations from the Centers for Disease Control and Prevention, the National Institutes of Health, and the HIV Medicine Association of the Infectious Diseases Society of America. Available at: http://aidsinfo.nih.gov/contentfiles/lvguidelines/adult_oi.pdf. Accessed May 25, 2017.

15. Nahid P, Dorman SE, Alipanah N, et al. Official American Thoracic Society/Centers for Disease Control and Prevention/Infectious Diseases Society of America clinical practice guidelines: treatment of drug-susceptible tuberculosis. Clin Infect Dis 2016;63(7):e147–95.

16. Centers for Disease Control and Prevention. Treatment for TB disease. Available at: https://www.cdc.gov/tb/topic/treatment/tbdisease.htm Accessed June 10, 2017.

17. Centers for Disease Control and Prevention. The ABCs of hepatitis. Available at: https://www.cdc.gov/hepatitis/resources/professionals/pdfs/abctable.pdf. Accessed June 10, 2017.

18. Centers for Disease Control and Prevention. Viral hepatitis serology training. Available at: https://www.cdc.gov/hepatitis/resources/professionals/training/serology/training.htm. Accessed June 10, 2017.

19. Terrault NA, Bzowej NH, Chang K, et al. AASLD guidelines for treatment of chronic hepatitis B. Hepatology 2016;63(1):261–83.

20. US Food and Drug Administration. Tenofovir alafenamide fumarate. Available at: https://www.accessdata.fda.gov/scripts/cder/daf/index.cfm?event=overview.process&ApplNo=208464. Accessed June 13, 2017.

21. University of California, San Francisco. 2013. Comparison of 2 tenofovir prodrugs: TAF and TDF. Available at: http://hivinsite.ucsf.edu/insite?page=hmq-1305-01. Accessed June 13, 2017.

22. US Food and Drug Administration. Descovy: emtricitabine; tenofovir alafenamide fumarate. Available at: https://www.accessdata.fda.gov/scripts/cder/daf/index.cfm?event=overview.process&ApplNo=208215. Accessed June 13, 2017.

23. Edlin BR, Eckhardt BJ, Shu MA, et al. Toward a more accurate estimate of the prevalence of hepatitis C in the United States. Hepatology 2015;62:1353–63.

24. Campbell CA, Canary L, Smith N, et al. State HCV incidence and policies related to HCV preventive and treatment services for persons who inject drugs — United States, 2015–2016. MMWR Morb Mortal Wkly Rep 2017;66:465–9.

25. Centers for Disease Control and Prevention. HCV FAQs for health care professionals. Available at: https://www.cdc.gov/hepatitis/hcv/hcvfaq.htm#section1. Accessed June 15, 2017.

26. American Association for the Study of Liver Diseases. HCV testing and linkage to care. 2016. Available at: http://www.hcvguidelines.org/full-report/hcv-testing-and-linkage-care. Accessed June 15, 2017.

27. Freeman AJ, Dore GJ, Law MG, et al. Estimating progression to cirrhosis in chronic hepatitis C virus infection. Hepatology 2001;34(4):809–16.

28. Poynard T, Bedossa P, Opolon P. Natural history of liver fibrosis progression in patients with chronic hepatitis C. Lancet 1997;359(9055):825–32.

29. Giordano TP, Kramer JR, Souchek J, et al. Cirrhosis and hepatocellular carcinoma in HIV-infected veterans with and without the hepatitis C virus: a cohort study, 1992-2001. Arch Intern Med 2004;164(21):2349–54.

30. Shahid I, AlMalki WH, Hassan S, et al. Real-world challenges for hepatitis C virus medications: a critical overview. Crit Rev Microbiol 2017. [Epub ahead of print].

31. Rajani AK, Ravindra BK, Dkhar SA. Telaprevir: changing the standard of care of chronic hepatitis C. J Postgrad Med 2013;59(1):42–7.

32. American Association for the Study of Liver Diseases. Initial treatment of HCV infection. Available at: http://www.hcvguidelines.org/full-report/initial-treatment-hcv-infection Accessed June 20, 2017.

33. American Association for the Study of Liver Diseases. Unique patient populations: patients with HIV/HCV coinfection. Available at: http://www.hcvguidelines.org/full-report/unique-patient-populations-patients-hivhcv-coinfection. Accessed June 20, 2017.

34. American Association for the Study of Liver Diseases. HCV guidance: recommendations for testing, managing, and treating hepatitis C. Available at: http://www.hcvguidelines.org/. Accessed June 10, 2017.

35. Naing C, Sitt T, Aung AT, et al. Sustained virologic response to a dual peginterferon alfa-2a and ribavirin in treating chronic hepatitis C infection: a retrospective cohort study. Medicine 2015;94(30):e1234.

36. Bauer M, Leavens A, Schwartzman K. A systematic review and meta-analysis of the impact of tuberculosis on health-related quality of life. Qual Life Res 2013; 22(8):2213–35.

37. Bauer M, Ahmed S, Benedetti A, et al. Health-related quality of life and tuberculosis: a longitudinal cohort study. Health Qual Life Outcomes 2015;13(1):65.

38. Marra CA, Marra F, Colley L, et al. Health-related quality of life trajectories among adults with tuberculosis: differences between latent and active infection. Chest 2008;133(2):396–403.

39. Kibrisli E, Bez Y, Yilmaz A, et al. High social anxiety and poor quality of life in patients with pulmonary tuberculosis. Medicine 2015;94(4):e413.

40. Singh SK, Agrawal A, Tiwari KK. Improvement in quality of life in pulmonary tuberculosis patients: a prospective study. Trop Doctor 2017;47(2):97–100.

41. Mthiyane T, Pym A, Dheda K, et al. Longitudinal assessment of health related quality of life of HIV infected patients treated for tuberculosis and HIV in a high burden setting. Qual Life Res 2016;25(12):3067–76.
42. Modabbernia A, Ashrafi M, Malekzadeh R, et al. A review of psychosocial issues in patients with chronic hepatitis B. Arch Iran Med 2013;16(2):114–22.
43. Karacaer Z, Cakir B, Erdem H, et al. Quality of life and related factors among chronic hepatitis B-infected patients: a multi-center study. Health Qual Life Outcomes 2016;14:153.
44. Keskin G, Gumus AB, Orgun F. Quality of life, depression, and anxiety among hepatitis B patients. Gastroenterol Nurs 2013;36(5):346–56.
45. Youssef NF, El Kassas M, Farag A, et al. Health-related quality of life in patients with chronic hepatitis C receiving sofosbuvir-based treatment, with and without interferon: a prospective observational study in Egypt. BMC Gastroenterol 2017;17:1–16.
46. Scheiner B, Schwabl P, Steiner S, et al. Interferon-free regimens improve health-related quality of life and fatigue in HIV/HCV-coinfected patients with advanced liver disease: a retrospective study. Medicine 2016;95(27):1–8.
47. Younossi ZM, Stepanova M, Estaban R, et al. Superiority of interferon-free regimens for chronic hepatitis C: the effect on health-related quality of life and work productivity. Medicine 2017;96(7):1–6.

A Therapeutic Perspective of Living with Human Immunodeficiency Virus/AIDS in 2017

CrossMark

David B. Cluck, PharmD[a],*, Roxanne F. Underwood, FNP-BC[b]

KEYWORDS

- Antiretroviral therapy • HIV/AIDS • Preexposure prophylaxis
- Antiretroviral drug-drug interactions

KEY POINTS

- Antiretroviral therapy has evolved since being introduced in the late 1980s with more effective and tolerable agents being available to clinicians today.
- Patients with human immunodeficiency virus are living longer and have a life span comparable to patients who are not infected, emphasizing the relevance of drug-drug interactions and managing comorbidities.
- Antiretroviral therapy is on the brink of significant change with long-acting injectable agents on the horizon.

CASE VIGNETTE

A 22-year-old man presented to the emergency department in October of 1995 with a 5-day history of myalgia, cough, dyspnea, and nonbloody diarrhea. He had been ill for several days, ultimately seeking treatment for increased shortness of breath and fatigue. He is diagnosed with *Pneumocystis* pneumonia secondary to AIDS. He is discharged several weeks later with a prescription for daily trimethoprim-sulfamethoxazole. He sees a local infectious disease physician who starts him on zidovudine, didanosine, and saquinavir.

Disclosure Statement: The authors have nothing to disclose.
[a] Department of Pharmacy Practice, East Tennessee State University, Gatton College of Pharmacy, Box 70657, Johnson City, TN 37615, USA; [b] Infectious Diseases, Quillen College of Medicine, East Tennessee State University, HIV Center of Excellence, 615 North State of Franklin Road, Johnson City, TN 37604, USA
* Corresponding author.
E-mail address: cluckd@etsu.edu

https://doi.org/10.1016/j.cnur.2017.10.009
0029-6465/18/

nursing.theclinics.com

INTRODUCTION

Human immunodeficiency virus (HIV) continues to burden patient populations across the world despite remarkable advances in antiretroviral therapy. This is perhaps best exemplified by the 2015 "Indiana outbreak" in Scott County, Indiana, which brought HIV back into national focus after incidence drastically increased over a very short period.[1,2] This outbreak illustrates the complexity of issues, beyond access to care, which facilitates the persistence of the disease in the United States. Without question, living with and managing HIV in the United States today is much different from what it was when drug therapy first emerged in 1987.[3] Newer, better-tolerated therapies have since become available, making a once-challenging and stigmatizing disease state more manageable from both a therapeutic and lifestyle perspective. This article reviews recent changes in epidemiology of HIV, outlines commonly used therapeutic options and management of comorbid conditions, and provides future direction of therapy for patients living with HIV/AIDS.

EPIDEMIOLOGY

According to the World Health Organization (WHO), by the end of 2015, approximately 36.7 million people around the world were living with HIV.[4] Globally, sub-Saharan Africa has the highest incidence of patients affected, with nearly half of all new infections originating in the region.[4] In 2014, there were an estimated 1.1 million persons living with HIV infection in the United States; this number includes the estimated 15% of those persons whose infections had not yet been diagnosed.[5] Despite this, the incidence in the United States has decreased nearly 20% from 2005 to 2014, thought to be secondary to reductions in heterosexual transmission.[6] Demographically, women in particular have had the greatest decrease in new diagnoses at approximately 40%.[6] Unfortunately, these data also revealed a continued trend of disproportionately impacted patient populations, specifically among Latino and African American men who have sex with men (MSM).[6] In 2015, nearly half of new HIV diagnoses were among African American individuals. More than half of the African American demographic diagnosed reported their risk factor as homosexual or bisexual contact.[7] Of these "targeted" populations, the predominance of new diagnoses appear to be geographically concentrated in the southeastern United States, with one epidemiologic study finding more than half of all newly diagnosed patients being from the South.[8] This was best exemplified by a recent surge of new cases of HIV in Jackson, Mississippi.[9] This is thought to be the result of a complex interplay among demographic, psychosocial, and socioeconomic factors.[10] Mortality is also higher in the southern states, paralleled and perhaps correlated by those unaware of their diagnosis. The continued burden on those affected by HIV across the United States as illustrated by the continuum of care cascade was ultimately the stimulus for the National HIV/AIDS strategy in an effort to "close the chasm" between patients who are diagnosed or are unaware of their status and linkage to care with subsequent virologic suppression. This is an oft-cited target, referred to as "90 to 90 to 90." By 2020, 90% of all people living with HIV will be diagnosed with the disease, receive sustained antiretroviral therapy, and achieve viral suppression.[11] Part of the focus with the "90 to 90 to 90" model is "TasP," or treatment as prevention, which emphasizes efforts of being placed on halting transmission of disease.

EVOLUTION OF ANTIRETROVIRAL THERAPY

Treating patients with HIV has taken monumental steps since the discovery of the virus in 1981. Initially, zidovudine was the only available agent and led to unacceptable patient outcomes as monotherapy. Slowly, other antiretroviral drugs and drug classes were introduced and eventually a combination or "cocktail" of drugs became the standard of care. With these combination regimens came tolerability and pill burden issues in addition to limited access to therapy due to cost.

Today, clinicians are able to select from several drug classes to construct an optimal patient-specific regimen. Currently there are 6 drug classes and nearly 30 different agents; however, some agents have become antiquated and yielded to newer, safer agents. **Fig. 1** provides an overview of drug targets associated with each class. More so than ever before, patients are able to be started on therapy, in some cases the same day as diagnosis, with only a single, well-tolerated tablet. There are numerous factors that must be considered when selecting a regimen for a particular patient. Perhaps the most important consideration in starting therapy is the ability for the patient to be consistently adherent to the antiretroviral regimen. Poor adherence influences development of resistance after exposure to antiretroviral agents. Other factors that should be considered include potential for drug-drug interactions, tolerability, and comorbid conditions.

In recent years there has been a change in guidelines regarding when to start patients on antiretroviral therapy. The most recent Department of Health and Human Services (DHHS) HIV guidelines suggest all patients be offered antiretroviral therapy due to the benefits therapy may impart on the overall health of the patient as well as public health.[12] The Strategic Timing of Antiretroviral Treatment (START) clinical trial sought to gain finality of optimal timing for initiation of antiretroviral therapy.[13] The study was ultimately halted due to an overwhelming benefit demonstrated in starting therapy, regardless of CD4 count. It is equally important to recognize that there are patient populations that may not benefit from immediate initiation of therapy, including hospice patients and patients with significant barriers to adherence, such as substance abuse or mental illness. Numerous studies have been published to address novel methods to improve adherence, including mobile phone reminders, integration of clinical pharmacists, and providing a financial incentive for patients to be adherent.[14–16]

Table 1 provides an overview of commonly used antiretrovirals, but notably does not list those agents that are no longer clinically relevant. When selecting and constructing a regimen for each patient, it is recommended to have at least 3 active agents in the regimen. As described later in this article, this can be more challenging

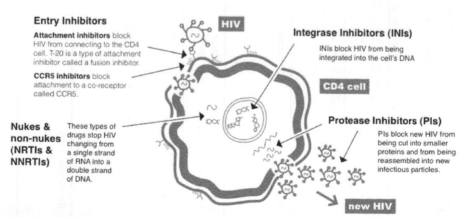

Entry Inhibitors

Attachment inhibitors block HIV from connecting to the CD4 cell. T-20 is a type of attachment inhibitor called a fusion inhibitor.

CCR5 inhibitors block attachment to a co-receptor called CCR5.

Nukes & non-nukes (NRTIs & NNRTIs) These types of drugs stop HIV changing from a single strand of RNA into a double strand of DNA.

Integrase Inhibitors (INIs)

INIs block HIV from being integrated into the cell's DNA

CD4 cell

Protease Inhibitors (PIs)

PIs block new HIV from being cut into smaller proteins and from being reassembled into new infectious particles.

new HIV

Fig. 1. Overview of drug targets associated with each class.

Table 1
Overview of commonly used antiretrovirals

Generic Name/Abbreviation	Trade Name	Dosing	Clinically Significant Adverse Effects	Clinical Pearls
Nucleos(t)ide reverse transcriptase inhibitors (NRTIs)				
Tenofovir disoproxil fumarate (TDF)	Viread	300 mg/d	Decreased bone mineral density; nephrotoxicity	Should be reserved for PEP, PrEP or pregnancy regimens
Tenofovir alafenamide (TAF)	Descovy Vemlidy (for HBV)	10–25 mg/d	Minimal	Available only as a coformulated tablet for HIV; attenuated effects on BMD and renal function
Abacavir (ABC)	Ziagen	600 mg/d	Hypersensitivity syndrome; associated with increased risk of myocardial infarction[35]	Requires HLA-B5701 allele testing to assess risk of hypersensitivity; diminished efficacy at viral loads >100,000 copies/mL[36]
Lamivudine (3TC) Emtricitabine (FTC)	Epivir Emtriva	300 mg/d 200 mg/d	Minimal	Active against HBV; avoid abrupt discontinuation in coinfected patients
Zidovudine (AZT)	Retrovir	300 mg/twice daily	Bone marrow suppression, headache, malaise	Only available intravenous ARV; utility in pregnancy/labor
Non-nucleoside reverse transcriptase inhibitors (NNRTIs)				
Efavirenz (EFV)	Sustiva	600 mg/d	CNS disturbances (vivid dreams, hallucinations); increased risk of suicidality[37]	Not recommended in patients with coexisting psychiatric disease; or new start in women of childbearing age
Nevirapine (NVP)	Viramune	200 mg twice daily (after once daily "lead-in" trial)	Rash	Increased risk of hepatic failure if used in men with CD4 >400 cells/mm^3 and women >250 cells/mm^{338}

Etravirine (ETR)	Intelence	200 mg twice daily	Rash	Retains activity against K103N mutation
Rilpivirine (RPV)	Edurant	25 mg/d	CNS disturbance, dyslipidemia (both less than EFV)	Lower efficacy in viral loads >100,000 copies/mL and/or CD4 counts <200 cells/mm[339,40]; requires high caloric meal for absorption Contraindicated with use of PPIs
Protease inhibitors (PIs) (used in conjunction with a pharmacoenhancer)				
Atazanavir (ATV)	Reyataz	300 mg/d	Hyperbilirubinemia causing jaundice, scleral icterus, cholelithiasis, nephrolithiasis	Should be taken with food to increase bioavailability; can be used safely in pregnancy; caution when used with acid-suppressive agents
Darunavir (DRV)	Prezista	800 mg/d or 600 mg twice daily	N/V/D	Caution in patients with sulfa allergy; should be taken with food to increase bioavailability; associated with a small, but gradually increasing CVD risk[41]
Lopinavir/ritonavir (LPV) coformulation	Kaletra	Four 200-mg/50-mg tablets daily	Diarrhea	Second-line PI, but has most clinical data in pregnancy
Tipranavir (TPV)	Aptivus	500 mg twice daily	Intracranial hemorrhage	Salvage PI; black box warning: intracranial hemorrhage
Integrase inhibitors (INSTIs)				
Raltegravir (RAL)	Isentress	400 mg twice daily or 1200 mg once daily	Skin reactions, new-onset depression	Well tolerated with few relevant drug-drug interactions
Elvitegravir (EVG)	Genvoya	150 mg/d	N/V	Available only as coformulated tablet; should be taken with food

(continued on next page)

Table 1
(continued)

Generic Name/Abbreviation	Trade Name	Dosing	Clinically Significant Adverse Effects	Clinical Pearls
Dolutegravir (DTG)	Tivicay	50 mg/d or twice daily if INSTI resistance present or suspected	Increased AST/ALT	Improved genetic barrier relative to EVG and RAL; recently associated with CNS effects in particular insomnia/anxiety[42–45]
Entry inhibitors				
Maraviroc (MVC)	Selzentry	150–600 mg daily depending on concurrent medications	Black box warning for hepatotoxicity	Requires Trofile to assess receptor profile (CCR5 vs CXCR4); caution with drug-drug interactions
Enfuvirtide (T-20)	Fuzeon	90 mg twice daily	Associated with increased risk of bacterial pneumonia[46]	Subcutaneous injection that requires reconstitution; associated with injection site reactions
Pharmacoenhancers				
Ritonavir (RTV)	Norvir	100–200 mg/d	Hypertriglyceridemia	Not to be used as a parent protease inhibitor; caution with drug-drug interactions
Cobicistat (COBI)	Tybost	150 mg/daily	Artificial increase in serum creatinine	Lacks antiretroviral activity; caution with drug-drug interactions

Abbreviations: ALT, alanine aminotransferase; ARV, antiretroviral; AST, aspartate aminotransferase; BMD, bone mineral density; CNS, central nervous system; CVD, cardiovascular disease; HBV, hepatitis B virus; HIV, human immunodeficiency virus; N/V/D, nausea/vomiting/diarrhea; N/V, nausea/vomiting; PEP, postexposure prophylaxis; PI, protease inhibitor; PPI, proton pump inhibitor; PrEP, preexposure prophylaxis.

in those patients who are extensively treatment experienced. In treatment-naïve patients, the guidelines universally recommend a 2-drug nucleoside/nucleotide reverse transcriptase inhibitor (NRTI) "backbone" typically composed of tenofovir alafenamide and emtricitabine (available as Descovy) in conjunction with one of the integrase inhibitors). Notably, outside the United States, WHO HIV guidelines recommend tenofovir disoproxil/emtricitabine/efavirenz (Atripla) for all treatment-naïve patients.[17]

In April 2015, the guidelines underwent significant changes regarding which regimens are preferred for treatment-naïve patients. **Box 1** outlines the preferred regimens according to the DHHS guidelines, whereas **Table 2** lists available combination antiretroviral agents. For the first time since its introduction in 1998, efavirenz is no longer recommended to be added to an optimized background regimen largely due to tolerability. Moreover, atazanavir boosted with ritonavir is now also considered an alternative PI-based regimen as a result of the findings of the AIDS Clinical Trials Group (ACTG) 5257 study.[18] Similar to efavirenz, the study revealed atazanavir-based regimens are limited by tolerability secondary to adverse effects. The integrase strand transfer inhibitors, now all considered preferred options, have gained widespread favor among clinicians due to their tolerability, limited drug interaction profile, and efficacy. The findings of the ACTG 5257 study, in addition to the changes to the guidelines, emphasizes the importance of the relationship between adherence and tolerability. The goal of initiating antiretroviral therapy is not only to improve the health of the patient, but also to prevent transmission. The HIV Prevention Trials Network (HPTN) 052, considered a landmark study, demonstrated patients on antiretroviral therapy reduced the risk of transmission by 96%.[19] The findings of HPTN 052 were reinforced by a subsequent study, the PARTNER study, which demonstrated zero linked transmissions among serodiscordant couples, with one partner achieving virologic suppression via antiretroviral therapy.[20] Together, these data highlight the possibility and efficacy of using a treatment as prevention strategy.

Although the "era of the integrase inhibitors" was ushered in with the newest iteration of the DHHS guidelines, changes to the NRTI backbone also occurred with the availability of tenofovir alafenamide. Compared with tenofovir disoproxil, this newer formulation has a significantly diminished impact on bone mineral density and renal function secondary to greater concentrations in lymphocytes relative to plasma.[21,22] In 2017, patients currently receiving tenofovir disoproxil should be transitioned to the newer formulation if for no other reason, safety. Despite this, tenofovir disoproxil and emtricitabine (Truvada) still has a role in caring for patients, as it remains the current recommended agent for use as preexposure prophylaxis (PrEP), postexposure prophylaxis (PEP), and in the treatment of women who are pregnant.

Box 1
DHHS preferred antiretroviral regimens

Abacavir/lamivudine/dolutegravir[a]

Tenofovir disoproxil/emtricitabine OR tenofovir alafenamide/emtricitabine plus dolutegravir

Tenofovir disoproxil/emtricitabine OR tenofovir alafenamide/emtricitabine plus raltegravir

Tenofovir disoproxil/emtricitabine OR tenofovir alafenamide/emtricitabine/cobicistat/elvitegravir

[a] Patient should be HLA-B5701 negative.

Table 2
Available combination antiretroviral formulations

Generic Name/Abbreviation	Trade Name
Abacavir/lamivudine	Epzicom
Abacavir/lamivudine/zidovudine	Trizivir
Abacavir/lamivudine/dolutegravir[a]	Triumeq
Tenofovir disoproxil/emtricitabine/rilpivirine[a]	Complera
Tenofovir alafenamide/emtricitabine/rilpivirine[a]	Odefsey
Tenofovir disoproxil/emtricitabine/efavirenz[a]	Atripla
Tenofovir disoproxil/emtricitabine/cobicistat/elvitegravir[a]	Stribild
Tenofovir alafenamide/emtricitabine/cobicistat/elvitegravir[a]	Genvoya
Tenofovir disoproxil/emtricitabine	Truvada
Tenofovir alafenamide/emtricitabine	Descovy
Zidovudine/lamivudine	Combivir
Atazanavir/cobicistat	Evotaz
Darunavir/cobicistat	Prezcobix

[a] A fully active single-tablet regimen.

Caring for treatment-experienced patients can be more challenging, as selection of therapeutic regimens is often driven by genotypic resistance in addition to degree of adherence and exposure history to other antiretroviral agents. Resistance manifests as point mutations conferring diminished activity against HIV. In turn, patients on regimens that have been compromised by resistance often will show a rebound in viral load after experiencing virologic suppression or lack of improvement in CD4 count.

Although resistance is most frequently a result of exposure to an antiretroviral, transmitted resistance also can occur and should be taken into consideration when selecting a regimen in treatment-naïve patients. Common mutations of clinical significance include M184V, which confers resistance to lamivudine and emtricitabine, as well as K103N, which confers resistance to first-generation non-NRTIs (NNRTIs) efavirenz and nevirapine. Moreover, transmitted resistance is particularly important for the NNRTI class, as it is most commonly transmitted in newly acquired infections.[23] Paradoxically, resistance to some antiretroviral agents can be beneficial. The aforementioned M184V mutation, commonly a result of selective pressure on drug initiation, can actually increase susceptibility of the virus to other antiretroviral agents.[24] Presence of the mutation also can have some impact on viral fitness.[25,26] Given that resistance and exposure to other antiretrovirals dictate management of treatment-experienced patients, particular characteristics of antiretrovirals, such as threshold to loss of virologic activity, commonly referred to as "genetic barrier," are also important in selecting a new regimen. Antiretrovirals, such as PIs and dolutegravir, have a high genetic barrier to resistance comparatively and are preferentially considered in nonadherent patients. Conversely, efavirenz and rilpivirine have a low genetic barrier and may not be appropriate for nonadherent patients. It is worth mentioning that data also exist using NRTI-sparing regimens in both treatment-naïve and treatment-experienced patients; however, results have been mixed and use of these regimens should not be routine.[27–29]

Finally, although efforts are ongoing to diagnose patients and get them into care, several clinics across the United States, as well as researchers, are placing increased emphasis on PrEP. This strategy is being adopted in an effort to prevent new infections in high-risk seronegative patients or serodiscordant couples. At present, the only antiretroviral agent approved for use as PrEP is Truvada (tenofovir disoproxil/emtrici-tabine).[30] Guidelines for candidates and subsequent follow-up are available through the Centers for Disease Control and Prevention and should be followed to ensure optimal outcomes are achieved.[31] Several studies have demonstrated efficacy; however, as with treatment, it is imperative that patients take the medication as prescribed. The IPERGAY study, boasting an efficacy rate of approximately 86%, is one example of how powerful PrEP can be in protecting patients without a high pill burden.[32] As mentioned previously, adherence is critical in these patients as well. Despite these findings, providers have been hesitant to prescribe PrEP for various reasons, including fostering resistance to the once most commonly used NRTI backbone, toxicities associated with tenofovir, and "behavioral risk compensation." To date, studies have failed to validate these concerns.[33,34]

AGING AND HUMAN IMMUNODEFICIENCY VIRUS

In 2017, data have emerged regarding life expectancy in patients infected with HIV. Patients who are virologically suppressed have been found to experience a similar life expectancy as those without HIV.[47] This exemplifies the impact drug therapy can have on patients, as well as just how far we have come since the days of zidovudine monotherapy.

The currently available therapies and the extended life expectancy of patients has resulted in an increased need for management of comorbidities, including cardiovascular disease, smoking cessation, and hyperlipidemia, as well as mental illness and substance abuse. Patients with HIV are at higher risk of cardiovascular disease through a complex interplay of biologic mechanisms and lifestyle choices, including chronic inflammation. Another plausible cause of cardiovascular disease is cigarette smoking, which is thought to be better correlated than any other risk factor. Although overall it is thought that smoking has decreased in the United States, more patients with HIV continue to use cigarettes. Recent data indicate patients are likely to experience reduced life expectancy secondary to cigarette use compared with HIV infection.[48] This finding should reiterate the need to counsel patients who continue to smoke to seek out smoking cessation strategies or at least be offered therapy at each visit. Dyslipidemia is also not an uncommon finding in the HIV patient population in conjunction with diabetes, thus also contributing to future risk of cardiovascular disease.[49] Despite this, most chronic disease states can be effectively managed with drug therapy; however, caution should be exercised to avoid polypharmacy as well as drug-drug interactions, particularly with statins. The management of both acute and chronic disease states has also heightened the need to be aware of drug-drug interactions for both prescription and over-the-counter therapies.

COMMON DRUG INTERACTIONS

Selection of antiretroviral therapy for patients is multifactorial, as described in the previous sections. Adding to this complexity is the possibility for drug-drug interactions. Certain drug classes possess a greater propensity compared with others to interact with other drugs largely due to their pharmacokinetic profile. Comparatively, PI-based regimens are particularly challenging, as they require ritonavir or cobicistat as a pharmacoenhancer. The purpose of the enhancer is to increase or "boost" the concentration of other antiretrovirals metabolized by cytochrome P450 enzymes; this lends itself to a plethora of other CYP-mediated interactions. With the relatively recent change to the guidelines and the introduction of several combination products containing another pharmacoenhancer, cobicistat, such as Genvoya (cobicistat, elvitegravir, emtricitabine, and tenofovir alafenamide), Prezcobix (darunavir/cobicistat), and Evotaz (atazanavir/cobicistat), this problem stands to continue to be clinically significant.

Several interactions warrant further discussion, as they are most likely to be encountered regardless of area of clinical practice. In some areas of the United States, hepatitis C virus (HCV) is highly prevalent, and treatment of coinfected patients is becoming more common. Patients who are coinfected can be at considerably high risk for relevant drug-drug interactions, given the pharmacokinetic profile of many of the newer antiviral agents. One of the most frequently encountered interactions was with Harvoni (sofosbuvir/ledipasvir) and tenofovir disoproxil. This interaction led to augmented concentrations of tenofovir disoproxil and risk of nephrotoxicity with the combination.[50] This risk has been mitigated with the introduction of tenofovir alafenamide. Antiviral regimens for HCV that contain PIs are more likely to have significant drug interactions with pharmacoenhancers.

Many patients today are currently prescribed or are purchasing over-the-counter proton pump inhibitors. These drugs are known to reduce the bioavailability of atazanavir and rilpivirine, with the latter being contraindicated with proton pump inhibitors. A significant number of patients are also receiving inhaled or intranasal corticosteroids, which are known to interact with pharmacoenhancers and are not recommended to be used concurrently.[51] This is routinely encountered in clinical practice, but perhaps easily overlooked given the local route of administration. Finally, many of the novel oral anticoagulants are not recommended to be taken concurrently with drugs that interact with CYP enzymes; however, dabigatran may be safe in some patients. Notably, warfarin, which interacts with known CYP substrates, should be closely monitored, but should not be considered contraindicated.[52]

FUTURE DIRECTION AND SUMMARY

Antiretroviral therapy has improved tremendously over the past 30 years. Although new agents are in the pipeline, more energy is being placed on efforts to prevent transmission, either through starting therapy or providing high-risk patients with PrEP, as well continued research in pursuit of a vaccine and/or cure. Moreover, data continue to emerge seeking ways to simplify therapy or make current treatment options safer. The recent findings of the SWORD study exemplify this strategy. The study demonstrated safety in simplifying patients to a 2-drug regimen using dolutegravir and rilpivirine while maintaining comparable virologic control to 3-drug or 4-drug regimens.[53] Despite a paucity of clinical data, many clinicians anecdotally have also used dolutegravir plus ritonavir-boosted darunavir given the exceptionally high genetic barrier both drugs share.[54]

The availability of newer agents on the horizon is likely to result in a paradigm shift regarding how both newly diagnosed and treatment-experienced patients are approached. These drugs include cabotegravir, a new injectable integrase inhibitor; bictegravir, an integrase inhibitor that does not require a pharmacoenhancer; and BMS-663068, an attachment inhibitor.[55–57] The long-acting injectable agents, cabotegravir and a nanoformulation of rilpivirine, also hold promise for use as PrEP.[58]

The patient in the case vignette demonstrates the tremendous progress made in caring for patients with HIV/AIDS today. Patients diagnosed in the late 1980s and early 1990s were considered to have a significantly shorter life span and subject to high pill burdens with inferior efficacy compared with currently available therapies. The antiretroviral regimens available to patients today are simplified and considerably less toxic and promote adherence while shattering common preconceived notions and myths regarding therapy. Initiation of antiretroviral therapy is more important today than ever, as there is not only direct patient benefit but a demonstrable public health benefit. With the introduction of newer agents, further therapeutic simplifications and continued access to care, living with HIV should no longer be the burden it once was.

REFERENCES

1. Centers for Disease Control and Prevention (CDC). Community outbreak of HIV infection linked to injection drug use of oxymorphone—Indiana, 2015. MMWR Morb Mortal Wkly Rep 2015;64(16):443–4.
2. Peters PJ, Pontones P, Hoover KW, et al. HIV infection linked to injection use of oxymorphone in Indiana, 2014–2015. N Engl J Med 2016;375:229–39.
3. Fischl MA, Richman DD, Grieco MH, et al. The efficacy of azidothymidine (AZT) in the treatment of patients with AIDS and AIDS-related complex. A double-blind, placebo-controlled trial. N Engl J Med 1987;317:185–91.
4. UNAIDS. Report on the global AIDS epidemic 2016. Avaialble at: http://www.unaids.org/en/resources/fact-sheet. Accessed June 15, 2017.
5. Centers for Disease Control and Prevention. HIV Surveillance Report, 2015. vol. 27. 2016. Available at: http://www.cdc.gov/hiv/library/reports/hiv-surveillance.html. Accessed June 21, 2017.
6. Centers for Disease Control and Prevention. Trends in U.S. HIV Diagnoses, 2005-2014. Available at: https://www.cdc.gov/nchhstp/newsroom/docs/factsheets/hiv-data-trends-fact-sheet-508.pdf. Accessed June 24, 2017.
7. Centers for Disease Control and Prevention. High-impact HIV prevention: CDC's approach to reducing HIV infections in the United States. Available at: https://www.cdc.gov/hiv/pdf/policies_NHPC_Booklet.pdf. Accessed June 27, 2017.
8. Southern HIV/AIDS Strategy Initiative. SASI update: the continuing HIV crisis in the US South: Duke Center for Health Policy and Inequalities Research (CHPIR). Duke University; 2012. Available at: http://southernaids.files.wordpress.com/2012/11/sasi-update-the-continuing-hiv-crisis-in-the-us-south.pdf. Accessed December 7, 2012.
9. Hurt CB, Dennis AM. Putting it all together: lessons from the Jackson HIV outbreak investigation. Sex Transm Dis 2013;40(3):213–5.
10. Aral SO, Padian NS, Holmes KK. Introduction: Advances in multilevel approaches to understanding the epidemiology and prevention of sexually transmitted infections and HIV: an overview. J Infect Dis 2005;191(suppl 1):S1–6.
11. UNAIDS. An ambitious treatment target to help end the AIDS epidemic. Available at: http://www.unaids.org/sites/default/files/media_asset/90-90-90_en.pdf. Accessed June 3, 2017.
12. Panel on Antiretroviral Guidelines for Adults and Adolescents. Guidelines for the use of antiretroviral agents in HIV-1-infected adults and adolescents. Department of Health and Human Services. Available at: http://aidsinfo.nih.gov/ContentFiles/AdultandAdolescentGL.pdf. Accessed October 18, 2017.
13. Lundgren JD, Babiker AG, Gordin F, et al. Initiation of antiretroviral therapy in early asymptomatic HIV infection. N Engl J Med 2015;373:795–807.
14. Shet A, DeCosta A, Kumarasamy N, et al. Effect of mobile telephone reminders on treatment outcome in HIV: evidence from a randomized controlled trial in India. BMJ 2014;349:g5978.

15. Saberi P, Dong B, Johnson M, et al. The impact of HIV clinical pharmacists on HIV treatment outcomes: a systematic review. Patient Prefer Adherence 2012;6: 297–322.
16. El-Sadr WM, Donnell D, Beauchamp G, et al. Financial incentives for linkage to care and viral suppression among HIV positive patients. JAMA Intern Med 2017;177:1083–92.
17. World Health Organization Consolidated guidelines on the use of antiretroviral drugs for treating and preventing HIV infection. 2014. Available at: http://www. who.int/hiv/pub/guidelines/arv2013/download/en/index.html. Accessed June 29, 2017.
18. Lennox JL, Landovitz R, Ribaudo HJ, et al. Efficacy and tolerability of 3 nonnucleoside reverse transcriptase inhibitor–sparing antiretroviral regimens for treatment-naive volunteers infected with HIV-1: a randomized, controlled equivalence trial. Ann Intern Med 2014;161(7):461–71.
19. Cohen MS, Chen YQ, McCauley M, et al. Prevention of HIV-1 infection with early antiretroviral therapy. N Engl J Med 2011;365(6):493–505.
20. Rodger AJ, Cambiano V, Bruun T, et al. Sexual activity without condoms and risk of HIV transmission in serodifferent couples when the HIV-positive partner is using suppressive antiretroviral therapy. JAMA 2016;316(2):171–81.
21. Sax PE, Wohl D, Yin MT, et al. Tenofovir alafenamide versus tenofovir disoproxil fumarate, coformulated with elvitegravir, cobicistat, and emtricitabine, for initial treatment of HIV-1 infection: two randomised, double-blind, phase 3, non-inferiority trials. Lancet 2015;385(9987):2606–15.
22. Gallant JE, Wohl D, Yin MT, et al. Efficacy and safety of tenofovir alafenamide versus tenofovir disoproxil fumarate given as fixed-dose combinations containing emtricitabine as backbones for treatment of HIV-1 infection in virologically suppressed adults: a randomised, double-blind, active-controlled phase 3 trial. Lancet HIV 2016;3(4):e158–65.
23. Ocfemia MC, Kim D, Ziebell R, et al. Prevalence and trends of transmitted drug resistance-associated mutations by duration of infection among persons newly diagnosed with HIV-1 infection: 5 states and 3 municipalities, US, 20062009. Abstract #730 in 19th Conference on Retroviruses and Opportunistic Infections (CROI) in Seattle (WA), March 58, 2012.
24. Whitcomb JM, Parkin NT, Chappey C, et al. Broad nucleoside reverse-transcriptase inhibitor cross-resistance in human immunodeficiency virus type 1 clinical isolates. J Infect Dis 2003;188(7):992–1000.
25. Campbell TB, Shulman NS, Johnson SC, et al. Antiviral activity of lamivudine in salvage therapy for multidrug-resistant HIV-1 infection. Clin Infect Dis 2005; 41(2):236–42.
26. Castagna A, Danise A, Menzo S, et al. Lamivudine monotherapy in HIV-1-infected patients harbouring a lamivudine-resistant virus: arandomized pilot study (E-184V study). AIDS 2006;20:795–803.
27. Raffi F, Babiker AG, Richert L, et al. Ritonavir-boosted darunavir combined with raltegravir or tenofovir-emtricitabine in antiretroviral-naive adults infected with HIV-1: 96 week results from the NEAT001/ANRS143 randomised non-inferiority trial. Lancet 2014;384:1942–51.
28. Stellbrink HJ, Le Fevre E, Carr A, et al. Once-daily maraviroc versus tenofovir/emtricitabine each combined with darunavir/ritonavir for initial HIV-1 treatment. AIDS 2016;30:1229–38.
29. Cahn P, Andrade-Villanueva J, Arribas JR, et al. Dual therapy with lopinavir and ritonavir plus lamivudine versus triple therapy with lopinavir and ritonavir plus

two nucleoside reverse transcriptase inhibitors in antiretroviral-therapy-naive adults with HIV-1 infection: 48 week results of the randomised, open label, non-inferiority GARDEL trial. Lancet Infect Dis 2014;14:572–80.

30. FDA approves first drug for reducing the risk of sexually acquired HIV infection. Silver Spring (MD): Food and Drug Administration; 2012. Available at: http://www.fda.gov/NewsEvents/Newsroom/PressAnnouncements/ucm312210.htm.

31. US Public Health Service. Preexposure prophylaxis for the prevention of HIV infection in the United States – 2014. A clinical practice guideline. Available at: http://www.cdc.gov/hiv/pdf/prepguidelines2014.pdf. Accessed June 29, 2017.

32. Molina JM, Capitant C, Spire B, et al. On-demand preexposure prophylaxis in men at high risk for HIV-1 Infection. N Engl J Med 2015;373:2237–46.

33. Lehman DA, Baeten J, McCoy CO, et al. Risk of drug resistance among persons acquiring HIV within a randomized clinical trial of single or dual-agent pre-exposure prophylaxis. J Infect Dis 2015;211(8):1211–8.

34. Mugwanya KK, Donnell D, Celum C, et al. Sexual behaviour of heterosexual men and women receiving antiretroviral pre-exposure prophylaxis for HIV prevention: a longitudinal analysis. Lancet Infect Dis 2013;13(12):1021–8.

35. Palella FJ, Althoff FN, Moore R, et al. Abacavir Use and Risk for Myocardial Infarction in the NA-ACCORD. 2015 Conference on Retroviruses and Opportunistic Infections. Seattle, February 23–24, 2015. [abstract 749LB].

36. Sax P, Tierney C, Collier A, et al. Abacavir-lamivudine versus Tenofovir-emtricitabine for initial HIV-1 infection. N Engl J Med 2009;361(23):2230–40.

37. Mollan KR, Smurzynski M, Eron J, et al. Association between efavirenz as initial therapy for HIV-1 infection and increased risk for suicidal ideation or attempted or completed suicide: an analysis of trial data. Ann Intern Med 2014;161(1):1–10.

38. van Leth F, Andrews S, Grinsztejn B. The effect of baseline CD4 cell count and HIV-1 viral load on the efficacy and safety of nevirapine or efavirenz-based first-line HAART. AIDS 2005;19(5):463.

39. Molina J-M, Cahn P, Grinsztejn B, et al, ECHO Study Group. Rilpivirine versus efavirenz with tenofovir and emtricitabine in treatment-naive adults infected with HIV-1 (ECHO): a phase 3 randomised double-blind active-controlled trial. Lancet 2011;378(9787):238–46.

40. Cohen CJ, Andrade-Villanueva J, Clotet B, et al, THRIVE Study Group. Rilpivirine versus efavirenz with two background nucleoside or nucleotide reverse transcriptase inhibitors in treatment-naive adults infected with HIV (THRIVE): a phase 3, randomised, non-inferiority trial. Lancet 2011;378(9787):229–37.

41. Ryom L, Lundgren JD, El-Sadr WM, et al. Association between cardiovascular disease and contemporarily used protease inhibitors. Seattle, February 13–16, 2017. [abstract 128LB].

42. Hoffmann C, Welz T, Sabranski M, et al. Higher rates of neuropsychiatric adverse events leading to dolutegravir discontinuation in women and older patients. HIV Med 2017;18:56–63.

43. Padilla M, Rojas J, Gonzalez-Cordon A, et al. Tolerability of integrase inhibitors in a real-life setting. 18th International Workshop on Comorbidities and Adverse Drug Reactions in HIV. New York, September 12–13, 2016.

44. de Boer M, van den Berk G, van Holten N, et al. Intolerance of dolutegravir containing cART regimens in real life clinical practice. AIDS 2016;30:2831–4.

45. Quercia R, Roberts J, Murungi A, et al. Psychiatric adverse events from the DTG ART-naive phase 3 clinical trials. Glasgow, 2016. Poster abstract P210.

46. Klein R, Struble K, FDA. Update to fuzeon (enfuvirtide) label regarding incidence of bacterial pneumonia. HIV/AIDS Update 2011. Available at: https://www.accessdata.fda.gov/drugsatfda_docs/appletter/2011/021481s020ltr.pdf.

47. Antiretroviral Therapy Cohort Collaboration. Survival of HIV-positive patients starting antiretroviral therapy between 1996 and 2013: a collaborative analysis of cohort studies. Lancet HIV 2017;4(8):e349–56.

48. Reddy KP, Parker RA, Losina E, et al. Impact of cigarette smoking and smoking cessation on life expectancy among people with HIV: a US-based modeling study. J Infect Dis 2016;214(11):1672–81.

49. Hadigan C, Meigs JB, Corcoran C, et al. Metabolic abnormalities and cardiovascular disease risk factors in adults with human immunodeficiency virus infection and lipodystrophy. Clin Infect Dis 2001;32:130–9.

50. German P, Garrison K, Pang PS, et al. Drug-drug interactions between anti-HCV regimen ledipasvir/sofosbuvir and antiretrovirals. In: Program and abstracts of 2015 conference on retroviruses and opportunistic infections. Seattle, February 23–26, 2015. [abstract 82].

51. Nelson B, Cluck D, Alexander K, et al. Need for awareness about interaction between nonprescription intranasal corticosteroids and pharmacokinetic enhancers. Am J Health Syst Pharm 2015;72(13):1086–8.

52. Egan G, Hughes CA, Ackman ML. Drug interactions between antiplatelet or novel oral anticoagulant medications and antiretroviral medications. Ann Pharmacother 2014;48(6):734–40.

53. Llibre JM, Hung CC, Brinson C, et al. Phase III SWORD 1&2 switch to DTG+RPV maintains virologic suppression through 48 weeks. Seattle, February 13–16, 2017. [abstract 44LB].

54. Capetti AF, Sterrantino G, Cossu MV, et al. Salvage therapy or simplification of salvage regimens with dolutegravir plus ritonavir-boosted darunavir dual therapy in highly cART-experienced subjects: an Italian cohort. Antivir Ther 2017;22(3):273–5.

55. Margolis DA, Gonzalez-Garcia J, Stellbrink HJ, et al. Cabotegravir + rilpivirine as long-acting maintenance therapy: LATTE-2 week 32 results. Program and abstracts of the 2016 Conference on Retroviruses and Opportunistic Infections. Boston (MA), February 22–25, 2016. [abstract 31LB].

56. Thompson M, Lalezari J, Kaplan R, et al. Attachment inhibitor prodrug BMS–663068 in ARV-experienced subjects: week 48 analysis. 2015 Conference on Retroviruses and Opportunistic Infections. Seattle, February 23–24, 2015. [abstract 545].

57. Sax PE, DeJesus E, Crofoot G, et al. Bictegravir versus dolutegravir, each with emtricitabine and tenofovir alafenamide, for initial treatment of HIV-1 infection: a randomised, double-blind, phase 2 trial. Lancet HIV 2017;4(4):e154–60.

58. Williams PE, Crauwels HM, Basstanie ED, et al. Formulation and pharmacology of long-acting rilpivirine. Curr Opin HIV AIDS 2015;10(4):233–8.

Stigma and Discrimination

Threats to Living Positively with Human Immunodeficiency Virus

Richard L. Sowell, PhD, RN, FAAN

KEYWORDS

- Human immunodeficiency virus • AIDS • Stigma • Discrimination • Positive Living
- Disclosure

KEY POINTS

- Over the past 2 decades, the number of individuals remaining healthy and living longer with human immunodeficiency virus (HIV) has increased dramatically.
- With the advancement of HIV treatment, individuals with HIV are living longer and enjoying a higher quality of health.
- If individuals are to have the opportunity to live positively with HIV, it will be necessary to challenge aggressively the beliefs and attitudes that result in stigma and discrimination against this population.

Thirty years into the HIV epidemic, we still have major discrimination and stigma related to HIV, as well as laws and law enforcement that drive people away from HIV services. Such situations are undermining the HIV response across the world. This will only change if we make major investments in programmes to reduce such stigma and increase access to justice for those affected by HIV.
—Michel Sidibe, UNAIDS Executive Director, 2011[1]

Over the past 2 decades, the number of individuals remaining healthy and living longer with human immunodeficiency virus (HIV) has increased dramatically. In addition, the number of new cases of HIV, AIDS-related deaths, and HIV infections in children has decreased globally.[2] These changes are a direct result of advances in treatment and the development and availability of more effective antiretroviral medications.[2–4] Despite such treatment advances, individuals with HIV continue to confront challenges to living positively, including being subject to stigma and discrimination. The following is a historical overview of the concept of stigma and an exploration of the causes and consequences of multilevel stigma for individuals with HIV. In addition, strategies individuals and societies use to manage stigma and avoid negative experiences are discussed.

The author certify that he has no outside funding or conflict of interest related to the article.
Academy of Inclusive Learning and Social Growth, WellStar College of Health and Human Services, Kennesaw State University, 520 Parliament Garden Way, Prillaman Hall, Room 4211, Kennesaw, GA 30144, USA
E-mail address: rsowell@kennesaw.edu

Nurs Clin N Am 53 (2018) 111–121
https://doi.org/10.1016/j.cnur.2017.10.006
0029-6465/18/© 2017 Elsevier Inc. All rights reserved.

UNDERSTANDING STIGMA

To understand HIV-related stigma, it is first necessary to examine the concept of stigma and its origins. Goffman[5] defined stigma as a characteristic or attribute that discredits an individual or a group. Society and its related culture establish what is considered normal or acceptable.[5] Stigma denotes a negative variation or departure from what are considered normal characteristics or attributes of individuals or groups. Variance from normal expectations often results in prejudice, discrimination, stereotyping, and distancing.[5,6] The ancient Greeks used the term *stigma* to refer to a sign or mark that was cut or burned into the body to indicate that the bearer was a slave, criminal, or traitor—that is, a blemished person who is ritually polluted and to be avoided, especially in public places.[5] In modern usage, the word usually refers to marks that are unseen.

Stigma and the negative responses to individuals thought to be different or unworthy—a phenomenon common in humans and animals—have continued over the centuries and across cultures and geographic regions. Individuals and groups can be stigmatized for a variety of reasons, including physical characteristics, ethnic or racial group membership, socioeconomic status, lifestyle, and medical conditions.[7]

Fear often underpins stigma. Individuals or groups who are perceived to pose a threat are targets for stigmatizing behaviors and negative actions. The act of stigmatizing an individual or a group allows and justifies actions such as discrimination, ostracization, and economic and social violence toward the stigmatized, actions that would otherwise be unacceptable. By stigmatizing the individual or group, it becomes acceptable to blame the individual or group for possessing the stigmatizing attribute, which in turn supports the concept of punishment for the stigmatized.[8]

HUMAN IMMUNODEFICIENCY VIRUS STIGMA

Not surprisingly, when HIV—a life-threatening illness with an unknown transmission source—was identified in the early 1980s,[9–11] it immediately invoked fear across society. From the start, HIV has been characterized by fear, stigma, and discrimination of people who have or are perceived as being at risk for contracting HIV.[1,7] HIV stigma results from a complex set of attributes, such as the fear of contracting a contagious, life-altering illness.[12] This fear often is overlaid with negative attitudes and beliefs toward groups or lifestyles thought to be associated with the disease.[12]

The fact that HIV initially was referred to as the "gay plague"[13] suggests early efforts by society to distance themselves from individuals at risk for HIV (gay men).[14,15] Furthermore, the term *plague* seemingly provided validity to the notion that HIV was a punishment from God for immoral or deviant behaviors.[16] These efforts also represent a case of *othering*, a process in which individuals subordinate certain peoples they perceived to be inferior in order to create superior identities for themselves.[17] The act of othering has been identified globally in many different cultures and is often based on racism, sexism, or homophobia.[12,18,19] Part of othering involves using behaviors and attitudes to distance oneself from the illness and its associated negative consequences and attributes, thereby supporting the contention that those individuals with HIV/AIDS are different from me.[7]

Causes and Double Stigmas

When members of one group are stigmatized for one reason, it is all too easy for society to stigmatize them further if they have HIV. First found in homosexual men, HIV later was discovered in Haitian immigrants, intravenous drug users, and people of color.[9,10] Individuals in these groups often were viewed as immoral and different from (less than) the rest of society and had been the focus of stigma and discrimination long before HIV was identified. In the United States, the highest rates of HIV are among men who have sex with men and African Americans, especially those living in the South.[20–22] These groups already were subject to stigma and discrimination before contracting HIV.

HIV stigma clearly is related to and exacerbated by other societal stigmas, including race/ethnicity, drug use, homosexuality, and poverty.[23] The association of HIV with groups that previously have been stigmatized helps establish negative attitudes and fear of these groups.[12,24] These negative perceptions of the disease and its associated groups are used as justification to discriminate against persons with HIV. Such actions likely would not have been as acceptable if these individuals had not already been stigmatized and devalued by society.

Parker and Aggleton[25] proposed that stigma and discrimination do not occur in a vacuum, but rather build on power and domination factors that underpin existing inequalities. Globally, the role of inequity and power relationships in the transmission of HIV and the discrimination associated with the disease are particularly observable in the overlay of HIV stigma with gender discrimination. Women, the aged, and the dying who have HIV also may face a double stigma. In some regions, women have limited rights and are considered the property of men.[26–28] It has been proposed that the continued spread of HIV in south Asia is the result of the trafficking of young girls into the sex trade.[29,30] In another part of the world, many African girls contract HIV between the ages of 15 and 19 years. In both of these examples, young girls become HIV infected because of sexual exploitation, gender-based violence, and economic insecurity.[31] In addition, the growing number of individuals living longer with HIV has resulted in a group of HIV-infected individuals who are growing older and having to deal with physical symptoms of both HIV and aging.[32–34] This phenomenon has added a new layer of stigma that is related to age discrimination.[35] In addition, being infected with HIV further added to the stigma many individuals with a terminal or chronic disease already experience. In Western countries where HIV treatment and prevention information have been available for decades, research demonstrates that even among health care professionals there remains a desire to avoid individuals with HIV infection.[36]

In contrast, even individuals without a double stigma still face HIV discrimination. Although those who contracted HIV through blood transfusions or exposure to infected blood products (including a large number of hemophiliacs) were not viewed as guilty or immoral, they still were discriminated against, because they had the mark of impurity.[5] In other words, individuals who previously were not members of a stigmatized group found themselves members of a newly stigmatized group: those who have the disease. HIV stigma has provided the underpinning that has justified neglect, physical and economic violence, abandonment, and subhuman treatment of persons with or believed at risk for HIV.

Consequences

In addition to having a profound impact on society globally,[37–39] HIV fear, stigma, and discrimination can have significant negative psychological and physical consequences for individuals, families, and communities. Research has demonstrated that HIV-related stigma and discrimination decrease quality of life.[40,41] Fear of stigma and discrimination also can result in a reluctance to disclose an HIV diagnosis.[42,43] Certainly, some individuals use nondisclosure or selective disclosure as a strategy to protect their well-being and quality of life.[44] Unfortunately, withholding HIV status or declining HIV testing can result in individuals not receiving needed treatment in a timely manner, which can have negative consequences for them and society as a whole.[45–47] Therefore, not only do HIV-related stigma and discrimination impact infected individuals' ability to live positively with an HIV diagnosis[7] but they also can negatively affect the trajectory of the HIV pandemic.

Governmental Involvement

As of 2013, 41 countries and territories continued to restrict the travel and ability to stay in the country of individuals with HIV.[48,49] Until 2010, the United States had similar restrictions.[50] In recent years, the United States and Canada have enacted legislative protections for persons with HIV.[51] Despite such protection, punitive sanctions or laws continue to affect persons with HIV.[52–55] These measures have resulted in HIV-infected individuals and the behaviors that put people at risk for HIV going underground, thereby decreasing access to treatment and prevention programs.[56–58]

A Continuing Problem

Despite advances in fighting the disease, HIV remains at pandemic levels worldwide and without a vaccine will continue to be a serious health problem.[59] Similarly, HIV stigma and discrimination remain a significant problem for those with the disease. Even in countries where access to advanced treatments has made HIV a chronic disease rather than a death sentence, HIV stigma and discrimination remain pervasive.[60–62] In resource-limited regions, individuals (especially women) with HIV can face physical violence, including the denial of access to life-saving drugs and medical care.[63,64] Although physical violence against individuals with HIV is rare in resource-rich countries, they still face rejection, ostracism, and economic violence.[30,65–67] Although some overt stigma-based behaviors have become less overt in recent decades, there remains an undercurrent of stigma that undermines the well-being and quality of life of many individuals with HIV.[68,69]

MANAGING HUMAN IMMUNODEFICIENCY VIRUS STIGMA AT AN INDIVIDUAL LEVEL

HIV-related stigma and the resulting discrimination can help create an environment in which individuals with HIV are challenged to maintain a positive quality of life. Strategies to address and/or avoid stigma occur on multiple levels. On the individual level, persons with HIV must assess their personal situation and environment to identify potential sources of stigma. This assessment and subsequent protective behaviors can begin with the decision to be HIV tested. Although HIV testing is considered the best HIV prevention approach,[70] individuals must consider the consequences of testing HIV positive before being tested. Important questions include the following: *Is the testing confidential?*, *To whom will the test results be disclosed?*, and *Are social and mental health resources available for those who test positive?* The ability to receive support and control the disclosure of an HIV-positive status can be the first steps in living positively with HIV infection.[71,72] However, research results indicate that a major reason preventing individuals from being tested and disclosing their HIV status is a fear of facing discrimination and being stigmatized.[73,74]

Disclosure

HIV-infected individuals use their level of disclosure to manage the degree of stigma to which they may be exposed. There are health benefits to disclosing HIV status to health care professionals who will provide treatment and care. The ability to maintain a high quality of life for many years is directly related to receiving the latest treatment and medications. Without disclosure, individuals will not have access to needed HIV treatment and care. However, some individuals disclose only to health care providers who have a need to know and are providing direct HIV care and treatment. In addition, depending on the state, persons with HIV may be required to disclose their HIV status to their sexual and needle-sharing partners as well as health care providers.[75]

The decision to disclose an HIV-positive status is a serious consideration that requires an evaluation of the potential costs and benefits of each disclosure. Such decisions need to be based on an individual's specific situation and needs. In addition to affecting the individual, disclosure can have serious consequences for family members and close associates. Women often are more concerned about the consequences of disclosure on their family, especially their children, than for themselves.[76,77] It also is important to remember that disclosure of an HIV diagnosis is not an all or nothing decision, but rather a series of decisions about how, when, and to whom to disclose.[7,78]

Research indicates that women with HIV may use specific criteria to guide their disclosure decisions. These 3 criteria are as follows: (1) their relationship with the individuals to whom they disclose, (2) the quality of their relationship with the individual (expectation of acceptance vs rejection), and (3) the likelihood of the other person keeping the information confidential.[79] Individuals with HIV may determine that full disclosure is not beneficial, but partial disclosure or disclosure to certain members of a group is necessary to support well-being.[78]

In contrast, some individuals decide to be open with their HIV status. Public disclosure can foster open dialogue within communities. Individuals with HIV sharing can help others relate to those living with HIV. Open dialogue in communities can facilitate understanding and help support a change in the social norms that demonize and discriminate against persons with HIV.[80] Health care and mental health professionals can play an important role in supporting individuals who want to disclose their HIV status to family members, friends, or the public. A 2-pronged approach, which supports HIV-infected individuals in disclosing their status and provides community HIV education, has the potential to help change attitudes about HIV and decrease the stigma and discrimination associated with the disease.

Religion and Spirituality

Although many individuals with HIV move away from formal religion due to prejudice against their lifestyle within the church, spirituality remains a positive resource for many individuals living with HIV. Religion and spirituality may have a positive effect on an individual's personal empowerment and coping abilities.[81] In addition, researchers have found that reliance on spirituality and religious beliefs among persons with HIV is associated with feelings that life is better.[81] Ironson and colleagues[82] reported that spirituality and/or religiousness increased in participants after HIV diagnosis, and this increase was associated with slower disease progression. Powell and associates[83] have recommended that churches and religious groups be more accepting of alternative lifestyles and support the health of all congregation members. This recommendation may be especially important for black churches because of the growing incidence of HIV and the importance of the church in black communities.[83]

Lifestyle Changes

To support positive living, individuals with HIV may decide to change their lifestyle and remove themselves from environments supporting the behaviors that put them at risk for HIV. A significant number of persons diagnosed with HIV have a history of substance abuse (alcohol and/or drugs).[44] For such persons, a decision to receive substance abuse treatment is a positive step in supporting their future quality of life.

Not only does this action alleviate the negative physical consequences of substance use but it also supports the individual's ability to adhere to medical HIV treatment. Individuals who do not have the resources to enter a treatment facility may turn to a 12-step program. Such groups provide an important forum for individuals with HIV to avoid isolation, interact with other, and learn how others are dealing with HIV.

Going Home

Another approach individuals with HIV use to remove themselves from environments that do not support their ability to live positively is returning to their families and communities of origin. In a study of older African American men in rural areas, Blake and colleagues[44] found that many of the men had moved from urban centers to rural communities. Men reported wanting to leave cities and the temptation to engage in negative behaviors in order to live a more peaceful life. One participant reported that being diagnosed with HIV had saved his life because if he continued the lifestyle he lived in the city, he would have soon died or been killed.[44] In this study, many of the men's identified health needs were related to dealing with advancing age and HIV.[44] In contrast, some individuals with HIV may move away from rural communities where the potential for stigma can be higher and maintaining confidentially is harder. These individuals may seek the anonymity of a larger city where they are not known and can live their life more positively with the support of others who are HIV infected.

ADDRESSING HUMAN IMMUNODEFICIENCY VIRUS STIGMA AT A SOCIETAL LEVEL

To end stigma and discrimination against individuals with HIV, both must be addressed at the societal level. There also is a need to address HIV stigma at the societal level to help individuals with HIV infections live positively within their communities. Researchers have suggested a variety of approaches. Avert presented a 4-part framework for addressing HIV stigma: protect, include, empower, and educate.[84] The concept of *protect* focuses on enacting antidiscrimination laws and decriminalizing HIV in order to challenge violence against individuals with and those thought to be at risk for HIV. The concept of *include* requires the redesign and implementation of health care services that facilitate the provision of unbiased HIV treatment and care while making stigma and discrimination reduction a national goal. The concept of *empower* supports individuals with HIV in understanding their rights and acting on violations to those rights. The final concept, *educate*, is designed to provide accurate HIV information that addresses the fear of HIV-infected individuals and changes negative societal attitudes about HIV.[84]

Another researcher contended that effective HIV programs address the basic causes of HIV stigma and provide inclusive HIV services that are available and accessible to those who need them.[80] Increasingly, there is an understanding that effective HIV programs include a human rights perspective and enlist individuals with HIV to help design interventions.[7,85]

Although we are still exploring what works, we already know what does not work. Stigmatizing individuals or behaviors leads to punitive approaches that have been shown to be ineffective and can compound the spread of HIV. Criminalization of drug use, sex work, and same-sex sexual relationships has failed to deter or eliminate these behaviors. In fact, public health analysis has shown that respecting individual rights and developing partnerships with HIV-infected individuals and groups at high risk of HIV infection offers greater effectiveness in reducing the spread of the disease.[1,73]

SUMMARY

It can be argued that access to health care and freedom from stigma and discrimination are basic human rights for all people, including those with HIV.[7] With the advancement of HIV treatment, individuals with HIV are living longer and enjoying a higher quality of health. If these individuals are to have the opportunity to live positively with HIV, it will be necessary to challenge aggressively the beliefs and attitudes that result in stigma and discrimination against this population.

REFERENCES

1. Joint United Nations Programme on HIV/AIDs (UNAIDS). Key programmes to reduce stigma and discrimination and increase access to justice in national HIV responses. 2012. Available at: http://www.unaids.org/sites/default/files/media_asset/Key_Human_Rights_Programmes_en_May2012_0.pdf. Accessed August 8, 2017.
2. Joint United Nations Programme on HIV/AIDs (UNAIDS). AIDS by the numbers. 2016. Available at: http://www.unaids.org/sites/default/files/media_asset/AIDS-by-the-numbers-2016_en.pdf. Accessed August 8, 2017.
3. Antiretroviral Therapy Cohort Collaboration. Life expectancy of individuals on combination antiretroviral therapy in high-income countries: a collaborative analysis of 14 cohort studies. Lancet 2008;372(9635):293–9.
4. Quinn TC. HIV epidemiology and the effects of antiviral therapy on long-term consequences. AIDS 2008;22(suppl 3):S7–12.
5. Goffman E. Stigma: notes on the management of spoiled identity. Englewood Cliffs (NJ): Prentice-Hall; 1963.
6. Jones EE, Farina A, Hastorf AH, et al. Social stigma: the psychology of marked relationships. New York: W. H. Freeman; 1984.
7. Sowell RL, Phillips KD. HIV/AIDS, stigma, and disclosure: a need for a human rights perspective. In: Holtz C, editor. Global health care: issues and policies. 3rd edition. Burlington (MA): Jones and Bartlett Learning; 2016. p. 261–86.
8. Abler L, Henderson G, Wang X, et al. Factors associated with HIV stigma in an urban area in China: results from the 2008 population survey. In: Proceedings of the XVIII International AIDS Conference: Rights Here, Right Now. 2010. Vienna (Austria), July 18-July 23, 2010. Abstract TUPE0565.
9. Centers for Disease Control (CDC). Kaposi's sarcoma and Pneumocystis pneumonia among homosexual men–New York City and California. MMWR Morb Mortal Wkly Rep 1981;30(25):305–8.
10. Centers for Disease Control (CDC). Pneumocystis pneumonia–Los Angeles. MMWR Morb Mortal Wkly Rep 1981;30(21):250–2.
11. Feller L, Lemmer J. Aspects of immunopathogenic mechanisms of HIV infection. SADJ 2007;62(10):432–4, 436.
12. Logie CH, James L, Tharao W, et al. HIV, gender, race, sexual orientation, and sex work: a qualitative study of intersectional stigma experienced by HIV-positive women in Ontario, Canada. PLoS Med 2011;8(11):e1001124.
13. VerMeulen M. The gay plague. New York Magazine 1982;52–78.
14. Health Resources & Services Administration (HRSA). Gay men and the history of the Ryan White HIV/AIDS Program. Available at: https://hab.hrsa.gov/livinghistory/issues/gaymen_1.htm. Accessed August 8, 2017.
15. Shilts R. And the band played on: politics, people, and the AIDS epidemic. New York: St. Martin's Press; 1987.
16. Sontag S. AIDS and its metaphors. New York: Vintage Books; 1998.

17. Joffe H. Othering of people and phenomena. In: Christie D, editor. The encyclopedia of peace psychology. Hoboken (NJ): Wiley on-line-Library, John Wiley & Sons; 2011.
18. Gilmore N, Somerville MA. Stigmatization, scapegoating, and discrimination in sexually transmitted diseases: overcoming 'them' and 'us'. Soc Sci Med 1994; 39(9):1339–58.
19. Petros G, Airhihenbuwa CO, Simbayi L, et al. HIV/AIDS and 'othering' in South Africa: the blame goes on. Cult Health Sex 2006;8(1):67–77.
20. Abbott LS, Williams CL. Influences of social determinants of health on African Americans living with HIV in the rural southeast: a qualitative meta-synthesis. J Assoc Nurses AIDS Care 2015;26(4):340–56.
21. Centers for Disease Control and Prevention (CDC). HIV surveillance report. 2017. Available at: https://www.cdc.gov/hiv/statistics/overview/. Accessed August 8, 2017.
22. Grey JA, Bernstein K, Sullivan PS, et al. Estimating the populations sizes of men who have sex with men (MSM) in US states and countries using data from the American Community Survey. JMIR Public Health Surveill 2016;2(1):e14.
23. Logie CH, Jenkinson J, Earnshaw V, et al. A structural equation model of HIV-related stigma, racial discrimination, housing insecurity and wellbeing among African and Caribbean black women living with HIV in Ontario, Canada. PLoS One 2016;11(9):e0162826.
24. Brinkley-Rubinstein L. Understanding the effects of multiple stigmas among formerly incarcerated HIV-positive African American men. AIDS Educ Prev 2015;27(2):167–79.
25. Parker R, Aggleton P. HIV and AIDS-related stigma and discrimination: a conceptual framework and implications for action. Soc Sci Med 2003;57(1):13–24.
26. Familusi OO. African culture and the status of women: the Yoruba example. J Pan Afr Stud 2012;5(1):299–313.
27. Mendenhall E, Muzizi L, Stephenson R, et al. Property grabbing and will writing in Lusaka, Zambia: an examination of wills of HIV-infected cohabiting couples. AIDS Care 2007;19(3):369–74.
28. Nwaebuni R. Nigeria: a difficult place to be widow. The Africa Report 2013. Available at: http://www.theafricareport.com/West-Africa/nigeria-a-difficult-place-to-be-a-widow.html. Accessed August 8, 2017.
29. Koler A. Sex trafficking and HIV/AIDS: A deadly junction for women. Human Rights 2010;37(2). Available at: https://www.americanbar.org/publications/human_rights_magazine_home/human_rights_vol37_2010/spring2010/sex_trafficking_and_hiv_aids_a_deadly_junction_for_women_and_girls.html. Accessed August 8, 2017.
30. Sarkar K, Bal B, Mukherjee R, et al. Sex-trafficking, violence, negotiating skill, and HIV infection in brothel-based sex workers of eastern India, adjoining Nepal, Bhutan, and Bangladesh. J Health Popul Nutr 2008;26(2):223–31.
31. Goldenberg SM, Silverman JG, Engstrom D, et al. Exploring the context of trafficking and adolescent sex industry involvement in Tijuana, Mexico: consequences for HIV risk and prevention. Violence Against Women 2015;21(4):478–99.
32. Ellman TM, Sexton ME, Warshafsky D, et al. A forgotten population: older adults with newly diagnosed HIV. AIDS Patient Care STDS 2014;28(10):530–6.
33. Centers for Disease Control and Prevention (CDC). HIV among people aged 50 and over. 2017. Available at: https://www.cdc.gov/hiv/group/age/olderamericans/. Accessed August 8, 2017.
34. Moore RC, Moore DJ, Thompson WK, et al. A case-controlled study of successful aging in older HIV-infected adults. J Clin Psychiatry 2013;74(5):e417–23.

35. Slater LZ, Moneyham L, Vance DE, et al. The multiple stigma experience and quality of life in older gay men with HIV. J Assoc Nurses AIDS Care 2015;26(1):24–35.
36. National Women's Law Center (NWLC). Health care refusals harm patients: the threat to LGBT people and individuals living with HIV/AIDS. 2014. Available at: https://nwlc.org/resources/health-care-refusals-harm-patients-threat-lgbt-people-and-individuals-living-hivaids/. Accessed August 8, 2017.
37. Bogart LM, Cowgill BO, Kennedy D, et al. HIV-related stigma among people with HIV and their families: a qualitative analysis. AIDS Behav 2008;12(2):244–54.
38. Hatzenbuehler ML, Phelan JC, Link BG. Stigma as a fundamental cause of population health inequalities. Am J Public Health 2013;103(5):813–21.
39. Mahajan AP, Sayles JN, Patel VA, et al. Stigma in the HIV/AIDS epidemic: a review of the literature and recommendations for the way forward. AIDS 2008;22(suppl 2):S67–79.
40. Fuster MJ, Molero, F. The relationship between HIV related stigma and quality of life among people with HIV. In: Proceedings of the XVIII International AIDS Conference: Rights Here, Right Now. Vienna (Austria), July 18-July 23, 2010. Abstract TUADO203.
41. Varni SE, Miller CT, McCuin T, et al. Disengagement and engagement coping with HIV/AIDS stigma and psychological well-being of people with HIV/AIDS. J Soc Clin Psychol 2012;31(2):123–50.
42. Akani CI, Erhabor O. Rate, pattern and barriers of HIV serostatus disclosure in a resource-limited setting in the Niger delta of Nigeria. Trop Doct 2006;36(2):87–9.
43. Visser MJ, Neufeld S, de Villiers A, et al. To tell or not to tell: South African women's disclosure of HIV status during pregnancy. AIDS Care 2008;20(9): 1138–45.
44. Blake BJ, Taylor GA, Sowell RL. Exploring experiences and perceptions of older African American males aging with HIV in the rural southern United States. Am J Mens Health 2017;11(2):221–32.
45. Lee SJ, Li L, Iamsirithaworn S, et al. Disclosure challenges among people living with HIV in Thailand. Int J Nurs Pract 2013;19(4):374–80.
46. Li MJ, Murray JK, Suwanteerangkul J, et al. Stigma, social support, and treatment adherence among HIV-positive patients in Chiang Mai, Thailand. AIDS Educ Prev 2014;26(5):471–83.
47. Mawar N, Sahay S, Pandit A, et al. The third phase of HIV pandemic: social consequences of HIV/AIDS stigma & discrimination & future needs. Indian J Med Res 2005;122(6):471–84.
48. Joint United Nations Programme on HIV/AIDs (UNAIDS). HIV travel restrictions: latest developments. 2012. Available at: http://www.unaids.org/en/resources/presscentre/featurestories/2012/july/20120722travelrestrictions. Accessed August 8, 2017.
49. Joint United Nations Programme on HIV/AIDs (UNAIDS). UNAIDS applauds Mongolia for removing restrictions on entry, stay, and residence for people living with HIV. 2013. Available at: http://www.unaids.org/en/resources/presscentre/pressreleaseandstatementarchive/2013/january/20130131psmongolia/. Accessed August 8, 2017.
50. Goosby E. Gearing up for 2012 International AIDS Conference. The White House: President Barack Obama. 2009. Available at: https://obamawhitehouse.archives.gov/blog/2009/11/30/gearing-2012-international-aids-conference. Accessed August 8, 2017.
51. Elliott R, Gold J. Protection against discrimination based on HIV/AIDS status in Canada: the legal framework. HIV AIDS Policy Law Rev 2005;10(1):20–31.

52. Centers for Disease Control and Prevention (CDC). HIV-specific criminal laws. 2017. Available at: http://www.cdc.gov/hiv/policies/law/states/exposure.html. Accessed August 8, 2017.
53. Chang F, Prytherch H, Nesbitt RC, et al. HIV-related travel restrictions: trends and country characteristics. Glob Health Action 2013;6:20472.
54. Lambda Legal. 2010. HIV criminalization: state laws criminalizing conduct based on HIV status. Available at: https://www.lambdalegal.org/publications/fs_hiv-criminalization. Accessed August 8, 2017.
55. Yager A. License denied: professional and vocational licensing restrictions affecting people living with HIV in the United States. In: Proceeding of the XIX International AIDS Conference. Washington, DC, July 22–27, 2012. Abstract TUPDD0102.
56. Molina E, Lainez H. Criminalization of sex work as an obstacle for access to integral attention on HIV/AIDS. In: Proceedings of the XVIII International AIDS Conference: Rights Here, Right Now. Vienna (Austria), July 18–23, 2010. Abstract TUPE1004.
57. Poteat T, Diouf D, Drame FM, et al. HIV risk among MSM in Senegal: a qualitative rapid assessment of the impact of enforcing laws that criminalize same sex practices. PLoS One 2011;6(12):E28760.
58. Joint United Nations Programme on HIV/AIDs (UNAIDS). International consultation on the criminalization of HIV transmission. 2008. Available at: http://data.unaids.org/pub/Report/2008/20080919_hivcriminalization_meetingreport_en.pdf. Accessed August 8, 2017.
59. Joint United Nations Programme on HIV/AIDs (UNAIDS). Global statistics. 2016. Available at: https://www.hiv.gov/hiv-basics/overview/data-and-trends/global-statistics. Accessed August 8, 2017.
60. Block RG. Is it just me? Experiences of HIV-related stigma. J HIV AIDS Soc Serv 2009;8(1):1–19.
61. Dlamini PS, Kohi TW, Uys LR, et al. Verbal and physical abuse and neglect as manifestations of HIV/AIDS stigma in five African countries. Public Health Nurs 2007;24(5):389–99.
62. Sengupta S, Strauss RP, Miles MS, et al. A conceptual model exploring the relationship between HIV stigma and implementing HIV clinical trials in rural communities of North Carolina. N C Med J 2010;71(2):113–22.
63. Dunkle KL, Jewkes RK, Nduna M, et al. Perpetration of partner violence and HIV risk behaviour among young men in the rural Eastern Cape, South Africa. AIDS 2006;20(16):2107–14.
64. Jewkes RK, Dunkle K, Nduna M, et al. Intimate partner violence, relationship power inequity, and incidence of HIV infection in young women in South Africa: a cohort study. Lancet 2010;376(9734):41–8.
65. Mukolo A, Blevins M, Victor B, et al. Correlates of social exclusion and negative labeling and devaluation of people living with HIV/AIDS in rural settings: evidence from a General Household Survey in Zambézia Province, Mozambique. PLoS One 2013;8(10):e75744.
66. Holtz C, Sowell R, VanBrackle L, et al. A quantitative study of factors influencing quality of life in rural Mexican women diagnosed with HIV. J Assoc Nurses AIDS Care 2014;25(6):555–67.
67. Ogunmefun C, Gilbert L, Schatz E. Older female caregivers and HIV/AIDS-related secondary stigma in rural South Africa. J Cross Cult Gerontol 2011; 26(1):85–102.

68. Anderson BJ. HIV stigma and discrimination persist, even in health care. Virtual Mentor 2009;11(12):998–1001.
69. Blake BJ, Taylor GA, Reid P, et al. Experiences of women in obtaining human immunodeficiency virus testing and healthcare services. J Am Acad Nurse Pract 2008;20(1):40–6.
70. Hayes R, Sabapathy K, Fidler S. Universal testing and treatment as an HIV prevention strategy: research questions and methods. Curr HIV Res 2011;9(6): 429–45.
71. Smith R, Rossetto K, Peterson BL. A meta-analysis of disclosure of one's HIV-positive status, stigma and social support. AIDS Care 2008;20(10):1266–75.
72. Vyavaharkar M, Moneyham L, Corwin S, et al. HIV-disclosure, social support, and depression among HIV-infected African American women living in the rural southeastern United States. AIDS Educ Prev 2011;23(1):78–90.
73. Abaynew Y, Deribew A, Deribe K. Factors associated with late presentation to HIV/AIDS care in South Wollo ZoneEthiopia: a case-control study. AIDS Res Ther 2011;8:8.
74. Duff P, Kipp W, Wild TC, et al. Barriers to accessing highly active antiretroviral therapy by HIV-positive women attending an antenatal clinic in a regional hospital in western Uganda. J Int AIDS Soc 2010;13(37):37.
75. HIV.gov. Talking about your HIV status. 2014. Available at: https://www.hiv.gov/hiv-basics/hiv-testing/just-diagnosed-whats-next/talking-about-your-hiv-status. Accessed August 8, 2017.
76. Nelms TP. Burden: the phenomenon of mothering with HIV. J Assoc Nurses AIDS Care 2005;16(4):3–13.
77. Walalu RN, Gill SL. "Living for my children:" mothers living with HIV disease. Southern Online J Nurs Res 2011;11(1):1–14. Available at: https://www.snrs.org/sites/default/files/SOJNR/2011/Vol11Num01Art03.pdf. Accessed August 8, 2017.
78. Bairan A, Taylor GA, Blake BJ, et al. A model of HIV disclosure: disclosure and types of social relationships. J Am Acad Nurse Pract 2007;19(5):242–50.
79. Sowell RL, Seals BF, Phillips KD, et al. Disclosure of HIV infection: how do women decide to tell? Health Educ Res 2003;18(1):32–44.
80. Macintyre K, Rutenberg N, Brown L, et al. Understanding perceptions of HIV risk among adolescents in KwaZulu-Natal. AIDS Behav 2004;8(3):237–50.
81. Szaflarski M, Richy N, Leonard A, et al. 2004 report on the global AIDS epidemic: 4th global report. Geneva (Switzerland): UNAIDS Joint United Nations Programme on HIV/AIDS; 2004. Available at: http://files.unaids.org/en/media/unaids/contentassets/documents/unaidspublication/2004/GAR2004_en.pdf. Accessed August 8, 2017.
82. Ironson G, Stuetzle R, Fletcher MA. An increase in religiousness/spirituality occurs after HIV diagnosis and predicts slower disease progression over 4 years in people with HIV. J Gen Intern Med 2006;21(suppl 5):S62–8.
83. Powell TW, Herbert A, Ritchwood TD, et al. Let me help you help me: church-based HIV prevention for young black men who have sex with men. AIDS Educ Prev 2016;28(3):202–15.
84. Avert. Stigma, discrimination and HIV. 2017. Available at: http://www.avert.org/professionals/hiv-social-issues/stigma-discrimination. Accessed August 8, 2017.
85. Barrett D. Track F rapporteur report. In: Proceedings of the XVIII International AIDS Conference: Rights Here, Right Now. Vienna (Austria), July 18-July 23, 2010.

End-of-Life Care and Bereavement Issues in Human Immunodeficiency Virus–AIDS

Karl Goodkin, MD, PhD*, Sindhura Kompella, MD, Steven F. Kendell, MD

KEYWORDS

• End-of-life • Death • Dying • Bereavement • Aging • HIV • AIDS

KEY POINTS

• Palliative care involves the evolution of a disease long-term, such that it presents with a comingled symptom burden due to the presence of multiple medical comorbid illnesses over time.
• Associated symptoms are not alleviated by the use of disease-specific medications and tend to persist, in many ways as indicators of chronic disease.
• Hospice care is care that supports the patient when the patient is imminently facing death and dying.

This article addresses 4 areas across the spectrum of end-of-life issues and applies them to human immunodeficiency virus (HIV)/AIDS: (1) palliative care, (2) hospice care, (3) death and dying, and (4) bereavement. An issue with this spectrum from the outset is one of definition: there is a frequent lack of appreciation for the differences between palliative care and hospice care. Palliative care involves the evolution of a disease long-term, such that it presents with a comingled symptom burden due to the presence of multiple medical comorbid illnesses over time. The associated symptoms are not alleviated by the use of disease-specific medications and tend to persist, in many ways as indicators of chronic disease. Hospice care is care that supports the patient when the patient is imminently facing death and dying. These 2 areas of care overlap, but their goals are distinct. In HIV/AIDS, in which premature aging is known to occur, patients come to palliative care earlier than is expected based upon the prior history of late stage referrals. This is a result of the dramatically successful development of the antiretroviral

Disclosure Statement: The authors have nothing to disclose.
Department of Psychiatry and Behavioral Sciences, James H. Quillen College of Medicine, East Tennessee State University, PO Box 70567, Johnson City, TN 37614, USA
* Corresponding author.
E-mail address: Goodkin@etsu.edu

(ARV) medication regimens for HIV infection. The former causes of morbidity and mortality have shifted primarily from complications due to immunosuppression to those characteristic of aging in the general population. Once hospice care in older persons infected with HIV has achieved its goals, then the care issues may move to the patient's experience of dying and, with the patient's death, on to the experience of the patient's death by others (bereavement). The hospice care stage also involves how a patient begins to mourn her or his mounting losses of functional capacities and, ultimately, to mourn her or his own passing in anticipation. Hence, each of the first 3 stages significantly overlaps, leaving the fourth stage of bereavement among the loved ones.

It has been more than 20 years since the advent of effective ARV therapy (ART), which was rapidly demonstrated to dramatically reduce AIDS-related mortality and morbidity in the United States.[1] In line with the long-term impact of those well-established treatment gains, it is anticipated that as many as 50% of persons living with HIV infection in the United States will be age 50 years or older by the year 2020. The causes of HIV-associated morbidity and mortality have melded with those of the general population, including coronary artery disease, myocardial infarction, cerebrovascular accident, neurocognitive disorder, diabetes, and cancer. Although HIV infection now may occur over an extended period of time, total physical and mental symptom burden eventually increase. Hence, the experience of HIV infection for the patient is eventually still converted to an experience in which there is a generalized expression of HIV disease progression (partly encompassed by the construct of frailty) that, to some extent, is not due to specific disorders that can be diagnosed and effectively treated. In line with these characteristics, the symptoms associated with this chronic disease burden are less likely to become the main focus of treatment attention by the primary care provider. Thus, there are several somatic symptoms associated with the longevity of HIV infection itself (or duration of HIV serostatus). These symptoms include fatigue, pain, insomnia, decreased libido and hypogonadism, deceased memory and concentration (HIV-associated neurocognitive disorder [HAND]), depression, and distorted body image. Palliative care for the chronic symptoms experienced by patients infected with HIV focuses on competent, skilled practitioners (effectiveness); confidential, nondiscriminatory, and culturally sensitive care (acceptability); collaborative and coordinated care (efficiency); flexible and responsive care (access and relevance to need); and fair access for all clients (equity). Palliative care has been associated with improved functional status in activities of daily living (ADLs), as well as with an improved quality of life for persons infected with HIV.

FATIGUE

Fatigue is among the most common and distressing symptoms associated with HIV/AIDS, affecting 20% to 60% of patients, and can be measured with the HIV-Related Fatigue Scale.[2] It is associated with increased release of proinflammatory cytokines, such as tumor necrosis factor-α, interleukin (IL)-1, and IL-6 from activated macrophages; and with clinical sickness behavior. The proinflammatory cytokines, in turn, are associated with increased HIV replication and with HIV disease progression. This cause of fatigue in HIV infection, among others, overlaps with causes of fatigue outside of HIV infection, especially in older patients. Common causes of fatigue include low testosterone levels, anemia, alcohol and substance use, insomnia, iatrogenic sources (eg, prescribed medication toxicities), obesity, diabetes, coronary artery disease, renal dysfunction, hepatic dysfunction, comorbid hepatitis C virus infection, and fevers of unknown origin. Other less common causes include cancer, chronic obstructive pulmonary disease, thyroid disease, and toxin ingestions. Of these, it is useful to note that anemia (particularly the anemia of chronic disease) is common in HIV infection, is an important cause of fatigue, and is a known risk factor for mortality in patients with HIV disease. Erythropoietin therapy is a safe treatment that is preferred to blood transfusions, improves quality of life, and may also (as a neurotrophic therapy) improve cognition and neuropathic pain (typically due to HIV-associated distal sensory polyneuropathy).[3] The symptom of fatigue in HIV infection should be addressed with a complete medical and nursing workup. Treatment should be offered for any specific, curable acute disease, as well as for fatigue that may be evaluated as due to a persisting identified disease (eg, hepatitis C virus infection), or for fatigue thought to be due directly to the HIV infection itself. Treatments for fatigue reported to have success with minimal side effects in those infected with HIV are modafinil and armodafinil.[4]

PAIN

Pain is a symptom that has been noted for some time to be under-identified and under-treated in patients infected with HIV.[5] The most common pain diagnoses in persons infected with HIV are: headache (46% of patients), joint pain (31% of patients), pain due to polyneuropathy (28% of patients), and muscle pain (27% of patients). One review of 61 studies showed that the prevalence of pain in subjects infected with HIV ranged from a point prevalence of 54% to 83% using a 3-month pain recall period.[6] The reported pain was typically of moderate-to-severe intensity, and pain was reported in 1 to 2.5 different sites. It is common for several different disorders to contribute to the experienced pain level of a patient infected with HIV at any given time. Moderate levels of pain interference with function were generally reported. All studies that reported on the adequacy of pain management recorded that there was a marked under-treatment of pain. Regarding treatment, it has been reported that HIV-infected persons more commonly receive opioids than HIV-uninfected persons.[7] However, patients infected with HIV received fewer days of opioids than uninfected patients and were less likely to receive long-term opioids. It is not possible here to address the complexity of pain management issues in this diverse patient group with multiple sites of pain on a chronic basis. However, it can be recommended that an effort should be made to develop pain management guidelines specific to the HIV-infected population because the data to date show that patients infected with HIV continue to be under-treated for pain, despite numerous studies published that document the frequent occurrence of pain in this population.

INSOMNIA

Insomnia is a common complaint in people with HIV and AIDS. One review reported that insomnia occurred in as many as 73% of out-patients with HIV infection.[8] Early studies reported sleep-specific electroencephalographic changes related to HIV infection, especially increases in slow-wave sleep; however, these results have not been confirmed by controlled studies since that time. Reports of insomnia are reported at all stages of HIV disease. Although insomnia is frequently reported as a side effect of effective ART, studies evaluating these medications have not demonstrated a significant effect, with the exception of efavirenz (found to be an independent predictor of insomnia[9]) and of raltegravir.[10] A large epidemiologic study of insomnia prevalence among persons infected with HIV demonstrated a high prevalence of insomnia (and daytime sleepiness).[11] However, persons infected with HIV did not have a significantly higher rate than matched HIV seronegative persons, although those data might be limited in generalizability to only HIV-infected persons who were diagnosed and treated early. Treatment is best initiated with non-pharmacological techniques, especially given the prevalence of concern for drug-drug interactions of psychotropic agents with ARVs in persons infected with HIV. Hence, treatment should begin with sleep hygiene, relaxation training, mental imagery, cognitive behavioral therapy (CBT), and self-hypnosis, as well as yoga and acupuncture.[12] If pharmacologic treatment is necessary, melatonin may be used without moving to prescribed agents. Among the prescribed agents, there is little to no HIV-specific randomized controlled trial (RCT) evidence available, though a variety of agents have been identified as first-line. These include very low-dose doxepin, mirtazapine, oxazepam, and zaleplon (for sleep-onset insomnia).[13] More recently, ramelteon (as a melatonin agonist) has been considered for this specific indication.

DECREASED LIBIDO OR HYPOGONADISM

A very common problem in HIV infection is the problem of decreased sexual drive and gonadal function. Moreover, the frequency with which this complication occurs in persons infected with HIV is compounded by the stigma persons infected with HIV face related to being active in their sexual interests. Low levels of testosterone may lead to fatigue, loss of libido, and dysphoria. Testosterone levels naturally decline with age, with about 20% of men older than 60 years and 50% of men older than 80 years having low levels of testosterone. In persons infected with HIV, overall 30% to 50% have low testosterone levels and the causes remain poorly defined. Testosterone replacement can be done by multiple routes (topical, injection, or oral). Each route has its own advantages and disadvantages. Testosterone replacement for persons infected with HIV has become widely accepted. However, recent reports have made testosterone replacement increasingly controversial.[14] Several recent studies have associated testosterone replacement with increased risk for cardiovascular complications. In fact, it has been suggested that testosterone replacement should be reserved, when possible, until additional, controlled studies of the efficacy and safety of testosterone replacement are carried out among the HIV-infected population.

DECREASED MEMORY AND CONCENTRATION (HUMAN IMMUNODEFICIENCY VIRUS–ASSOCIATED NEUROCOGNITIVE DISORDERS)

Decreased memory and concentration (and neurocognitive impairment [NCI], more generally) can occur in any stage of HIV disease but are most commonly seen in late-stage disease or AIDS. Currently, HAND is reported to occur in approximately 50% of persons infected with HIV in the United States on stable, effective ART. Of note, NCI may be the first symptom of AIDS in 10% or more of patients. The Frascati conference redefined HAND to be comprised by 3 categories: asymptomatic NCI (ANI), mild neurocognitive disorder (MND), and HIV-associated dementia (HAD).[15] ANI is a condition (not a disorder) and occurs when there is significant decline in 2 or more domains of neurocognitive performance assessed by standardized testing with no significant decline in ADLs. It is estimated that ANI (unlike MND and HAD) has not significantly declined in prevalence in the era of effective ART. For MND, there must be mild NCI in at least 2 domains of cognitive performance and mild functional impairment in ADLs. For HAD, there must be moderate-to-severe NCI in 2 or more domains of cognitive performance accompanied by at least moderate impairment in ADLs due to the NCI. Further, HAD is an AIDS-defining clinical diagnosis.

It has been documented that screening for HAND is not accomplished well by the widely used Mini-Mental State Examination, which is focused on cortical deficits rather than the subcortical deficits more prominent in HAND. Likewise, the Montreal Cognitive Assessment screening test, which is useful in the general population for minor cognitive impairment, has not been documented to be highly useful for HAND.[16] Evidence suggests that HIV-specific screening tests remain useful, including the HIV Dementia Scale,[17] though this test has been found to be lacking in sensitivity at lower levels of impairment, as well as to be culturally delimited. The International HIV Dementia Scale[18] is culture-fair and has somewhat greater evidence supporting its ongoing use in the era of effective ART.[19,20] However, current HIV-specific screening tests might well need to add selected, formal neuropsychological tests to optimize the screening accuracy for the presence and severity of HAND. Although formal neurocognitive testing at screening is not feasible, it is worth noting that patients may be screened with a self-report measure while waiting for their clinic appointments, using the Medical Outcomes Study HIV cognitive functioning scale,[21] though self-report tests are limited when compared with tests that objectively assess cognitive function.

The diagnosis of HAND demands a thorough medical and nursing workup because it is a diagnosis of exclusion. The workup should include a CT scan or MRI of the brain to rule out other causes of NCI, as well as a lumbar puncture (to rule out other causes and to generate a CSF HIV-load test). Metabolic causes and toxicity of alcohol, psychoactive substances, and prescribed medications must also be ruled out. Regarding treatment, reducing the impact of treatable, comorbid medical and nursing as well as psychiatric and mental health nursing conditions is a useful place to start, such as diabetes, hypertension, chronic pain, depressive disorders, and alcohol and substance use disorders. Second, the use of non-pharmacological methods should be evaluated, such as physical exercise and mental exercise, as well as formal cognitive rehabilitation techniques. Teaching patients to make and use lists and to use electronic reminders, as well as to use homework assignments on web sites displaying cognitive exercises, are all helpful in translating the insights from the clinic on specific cognitive deficits into improvements in a patient's ADLs. Third, pharmacotherapy may be indicated, with the use of central nervous system–penetrating effective ART regimens and psychostimulants being most generally recommended.[22]

DEPRESSION

Depression is a nonspecific term with multiple potential meanings. The most common representation is as a level of depressed mood, which everyone experiences in everyday life. However, it also represents a whole spectrum of disorders in which depressed mood co-occurs with a constellation of associated symptoms and is severe and consistent enough to affect ADLs; for example, major depressive disorder (MDD). MDD occurs at greater than 3 times the rate of the general population in persons infected with HIV.[23] Depression can also refer to adjustment disorder with depressed mood, dysthymia, substance-induced depressive disorder, and other related syndromes. When an HIV-infected patient who has not yet experienced any symptoms of HIV infection experiences her or his first symptom recognized to be related to HIV, she or he can no longer believe that HIV will never cause illness, dysfunction, and death. The ensuing general uncertainty about one's own health status is associated with an increased frequency of depressive spectrum disorders-more importantly than depressed mood level taken alone. The patient must learn to cope with this new uncertainty. It is important to be aware that the manifestations of depressive disorders may be confused with those of HAND or, in reality, depressive spectrum disorders and HAND may be co-occuring despite the fact that the diagnostic criteria for HAND do not allow for comorbid depressive disorders because of their confounding impact on neurocognitive function.[15]

Regarding the impact on HIV infection itself, MDD may be treated with the same medications that would be indicated for MDD outside of HIV infection. However, important considerations are side-effect profiles and the potential for drug-drug inter-actions. Of the selective serotonin reuptake inhibitors, paroxetine, which may also treat HAND,[24] and citalopram have been favored. Fluoxetine is best avoided because of its long half-life and the longer half-life of its primary metabolite (norfluoxetine) and because of its metabolism on both the CYP P450 2D6 and 3A4 isoenzyme systems. Of relevance to drug-drug interactions, these isoenzyme systems are also used by the ARVs. Bupropion in its higher dose range should also be avoided due to its dose-dependent seizure diathesis combined with that of HIV infection of brain itself.

It is also relevant to note that MDD has long been known to be associated with immu-nosuppressive effects in persons with HIV infection. MDD has been associated with decreased natural killer activity, as well with increased CD8+ T cell activation in HIV-infected women.[25] In numerous studies of MDD, MDD has been found to be associated with increased production of pro-inflammatory cytokines that are secreted by acti-vated macrophages in persons with HIV infection. This relationship provides a potential ground for a true synergism between MDD and HIV infection on clinical inflammatory outcomes, which are currently a prominent concern due to higher inflammation-mediated causes (rather than immunosuppression-mediated causes) of morbidity and mortality among HIV-infected patients with long-term suppression of plasma viral load on effective ART regimens. Martinez and colleagues[26] reported on a prospective cohort of 504 HIV-infected individuals initiating their first ART regimen in rural Uganda and found that higher levels of depressive symptoms were associated with both lower levels of plasma tryptophan and a higher plasma kynurenine-tryptophan ratio over 12-month follow-up. In contrast, declines in the kynurenine-tryptophan ratio and in-creases in plasma tryptophan levels partially explained effective ART-mediated im-provements in depressive symptom severity in that study. An increased production of 3-OH-kynurenine or quinolinic acid (formed later in the kynurenine pathway), or both, is found in persons infected with HIV. Relatively low levels of 3-OH-kynurenine can cause neurotoxicity by inducing oxidative stress and neuronal apoptosis. After interaction with cellular xanthine oxidase, 3-OH-kynurenine produces reactive oxygen species (eg, superoxide radicals) that cause internucleosomal DNA cleavage and, ulti-mately, cell death through apoptosis. Overproduction of reactive oxygen species has been associated with MDD. In addition, quinolinic acid is a potent N-methyl-D-aspar-tate receptor agonist. Intra-hippocampal injection of quinolinic acid in rats is known to cause substantial loss of hippocampal neurons. This links the overproduction of qui-nolinic acid directly with the hippocampal atrophy observed in MDD. Hence, MDD-associated impacts on inflammation could well play a role in the determination of the clinical outcomes of effective ART among persons infected with HIV.

DISTORTED BODY IMAGE

With the advent of the era of effective ART, a toxicity that soon became apparent was the lipodystrophy syndrome, initially termed "Crix belly" after the early protease inhib-itor ARV, indinavir (Crixivan). Lipodystrophy remains an incompletely understood condition characterized by a combination of central fat accumulation, peripheral fat depletion, and metabolic disturbances. An early study of HIV-infected heterosexual women and men who have sex with men (MSMs) with lipodystrophy syndrome showed erosion of self-image and self-esteem, problems in social and sexual rela-tions, threats to locus of control, forced HIV disclosure, demoralization, and depressed mood.[27] Relevant well-validated instruments are the Body Image Quality of Life Scale and the Situational Inventory of Body Image Dysphoria. They have been successfully used to measure body image effects. Self-reports of decreased facial fat and sunken cheeks were associated with lower infraorbital, buccal, and submandibular skin folds; a self-report of a buffalo hump was associated with a greater neck circumference; and a self-report of abdominal enlargement was associated with increased waist circumference.[28] Men were most commonly affected by lipoatrophy and women by lipohypertrophy.

Regarding treatment, non-pharmacological means can be effectively used first. A recent 2-arm RCT (n = 44) comparing CBT for body image and self-care with an enhanced treatment-as-usual condition at 3 and 6 months after baseline showed, at 3 months, that the CBT condition demonstrated substantial improvement in body image disturbance, depressed mood level, and ARV adherence.[29] The results were generally maintained, or improved, at 6 months. Regarding pharmacologic treatment, RCTs of switching specific ARVs have not had favorable effects on the volume of abdominal adipose tissue. Several small studies of lifestyle interventions, such as supervised aerobic and progressive resistance training, have reported modest-to-no reductions in abdominal adipose tissue but have yielded some improvements in associated metabolic abnormalities. Although these trials have been disappointing, lifestyle interventions are safe and appropriate to recommend as general health measures for patients with lipohypertrophy. The data do not support recommending metformin as a specific treatment of lipohypertrophy, although it may be used for abnormal glucose homeostasis in patients with lipohypertrophy who have impaired fasting glucose, impaired glucose tolerance, or type 2 diabetes mellitus, and mild or no lipoatrophy.[30] Similarly, testosterone repletion is not indicated solely to improve body composition in this population. However, recombinant human growth hormone (rhGH) has been used to treat AIDS-related wasting and is known to be lipolytic. Supraphysiologic doses of rhGH reduced visceral adipose tissue by 17% to 20% and improved lipid profiles in placebo-controlled trials in HIV-infected patients with abdominal obesity. The most promising intervention for lipohypertrophy is tesamorelin, a synthetic analogue of growth hormone-releasing hormone that yields more physiologic levels of insulin-like growth factor-1 than high-dose rhGH due to preservation of the negative feedback loop at the level of the pituitary. Two phase III, placebo-controlled trials of approximately 400 subjects per study have reported 11% to 15% reductions in visceral adipose tissue at 6 months in the tesamorelin arms.

In HIV lipoatrophy, a metaanalysis of 6 placebo-controlled trials found that pioglitazone therapy was more effective than placebo for increasing limb fat mass, but rosiglitazone was not significantly more effective. A meta-analysis of 16 trials concluded that rosiglitazone should not be used in HIV-associated lipodystrophy. Pioglitazone was also reported to be safer, but any benefits seemed to be small. Metformin was the only insulin-sensitizer to demonstrate beneficial effects on insulin resistance, lipids, and body fat redistribution.[31]

A variety of plastic surgery procedures have also been used.[32] For lipoatrophy, free flaps, lipotransfer, or commercial fillers or implants have been used to replace adipose tissue. Types of dermal fillers include poly-L-lactic acid (PLLA; Sculptra Galderma Labs, Ft. Worth, TX), a semipermanent injectable filler; polymethylmethacrylate (PMMA), consisting of 80% bovine dermal collagen plus 20% PMMA microspheres; and calcium hydroxyapatite (CaHA; Radiesse, Merz Aesthetics, Raleigh, NC), a soft-tissue filler consisting of 30% calcium hydroxyapatite microspheres and 30% carboxymethylcellulose. A 5-year study has shown that a polyacrylamide hydrogel-based filler is a safe and effective treatment of facial wasting. Other filler options include injectable bovine and human collagens, hyaluronic acid, and autologous free fat transfer. Further research is required to fully understand the psychosocial impact of lipodystrophy and to develop strategies that help individuals cope.

HOSPICE CARE FOR PERSONS INFECTED WITH HUMAN IMMUNODEFICIENCY VIRUS

The focus of this review thus far has been on how palliative care could be approached simultaneously with primary medical and nursing therapies aimed at long-term disease control and a functional cure in HIV disease. However, there comes a point in the trajectory of HIV disease progression in which palliative care begins to overlap with hospice care more than with primary medical and nursing care. In palliative care, the approach is to improve the quality of life of patients and their families facing the problems associated with life-threatening HIV disease progression through the prevention and relief of suffering by means of early identification, assessment, and treatment of pain and other symptoms, as well as other aspects of symptom burden (psychological and spiritual). In hospice care, the focus is on the end of life. Thus, the seesaw swinging up to palliative care from primary medical and nursing care converts to a new seesaw in which there is a swing up to hospice care from palliative care over time.

The stage of hospice care is one in which patients are provided with support to enter into the death and dying process (generally with a prognosis of 6 months or fewer to live).[33] Before the introduction of the ARVs with zidovudine (azidothymidine) monotherapy in the late 1980s, hospice care in HIV/AIDS was routine, though it also addressed the palliation of symptoms and provision of comfort for patients. With the subsequent evolution of ART into the dual nucleoside reverse transcriptase inhibitor therapy (NRTI) era, followed by the early era of highly active ART (HAART), a shift occurred in the care from dying with HIV/AIDS to living with HIV/AIDS. Thus, the move away from hospice-based care grew rapidly to the point that this form of care came to be perceived as irrelevant in HIV/AIDS. With the more recent growth of HIV prevalence in the older population, the acceptance of the need for hospice care of the HIV-infected has re-emerged.[34] Currently, an interplay between palliative care and hospice care is more relevant than ever before. Health care providers must use a truly multidisciplinary (rather than a multiple discipline) integration of knowledge to align and realign between a focus on a goal of primary medical and nursing care (and functional cure) of HIV/AIDS versus focusing on the goal of caring for the patient in need of symptom palliation and a later focus on anticipation of death and dying. The entire process occurs together with the need to plan with the patient and her or his loved ones for an increasingly uncertain future that continuously seems to waiver between a disposition toward an appropriately targeted, longer-term medical and nursing management approach versus a more intense, shorter-term caretaking approach. To a large extent, this shifting process of care is mediated by the variable impact of the aging process over time.

THE PROCESS OF DEATH AND DYING

As the pendulum of HIV disease progression shifts more regularly toward hospice care, the predominant clinical focus eventually becomes entry into the process of death and dying. This is the stage of the disease in which isolation of the patient from others both occurs more frequently, due to lack of comfort with the death and dying process by others, and it is most keenly felt. Ongoing assessments of spiritual well-being and meaning are integral to the death and dying process. Facilitation of this process requires being present; listening actively; assisting with advanced care planning needs (which should begin in early HIV disease); providing support for a patient's delineation of her or his desires; and guiding the patient, family, and other loved ones through the death and dying process. Although the stage of palliative care might be considered complete at this point, the needs of HIV-infected persons for symptom palliation persist throughout the illness to the time of death. However, it is true that it is the stage of hospice care that predominates here and carries forward the process to the stage of imminent death. Thus begins the stage of death and dying, a phase of the evolution of medical and nursing care that remains far too frequently overlooked today in HIV/AIDS.

An unusual, recent study of this phase took a phenomenological approach to the research participants in sharing their living experiences in confronting death and dying through storytelling.[35] Qualitative analytical methods were used to uncover 3 common narrative themes in this phase: making choices, transformation of fear, and meaning in death. The fear of dying was noted to be transformed into an energy directed toward living, while being cognizant that death remains present as a part of what defines life.

It has been more than 20 years since life-saving combination ARV treatments became available. The life expectancy among the subset of people living with HIV infection who had optimal therapy initiated early is now close to that of the general population. Worldwide, 1 million (830,000–1.2 million) people died from AIDS-related illnesses in 2016. In the United States, 6,721 people died from HIV/AIDS in 2014, and HIV/AIDS was the eighth leading cause of death for those aged 25 to 34 years and the ninth for those aged 35 to 44 years. Late diagnosis remains a key issue.[36] Meanwhile, UNAIDS (the Joint United Nations Program on HIV and AIDS) has set highly ambitious treatment targets for all countries: by 2020, governments will commit to ensuring that in any key population 90% of people living with HIV will know their HIV status, 90% of people with diagnosed HIV infection will receive sustained effective ART, and 90% of people receiving effective ART will have durable viral suppression. Although these are laudable goals to strive for at the population level, at the individual level it is important to recognize that people continue to die from HIV/AIDS in the United States, and much more so worldwide.

BEREAVEMENT

Beyond the death and dying stage of HIV/AIDS lies the emptiness left in the lives of those left behind by the deceased patient. This stage, the loss of the deceased patient (bereavement), is not generally included in studies done on the patient with a lethal complication of HIV/AIDS or HIV-associated non-AIDS conditions. Rather, it is considered outside of this scope because it relates to the loved ones of the patient rather than the patient herself or himself. However, bereavement is a potent life stressor with demonstrated chronic impacts on associated psychological distress (grief), neuroendocrine measures, immunologic status, and physical and mental clinical health status.[37] Because bereavement is no longer a frequent life stressor among HIV-seropositive persons, these effects have lost their former noteworthy focus of study in the literature. Yet, bereavement in the setting of HIV/AIDS still does occur and remains tremendously impactful.[38]

Research differentiating grief from depressed and anxious mood showed an 18% prevalence of unresolved grief in HIV-positive and HIV-negative MSMs.[39] Psychological distress is quite common in the year following loss.[40] Various time periods have been examined with respect to the development of complicated grief disorders. In fact, periods of 2, 4, 6, and 8 weeks, as well as periods of 6, 12, and 14 months, have been used. Despite this wide span of time examined after loss, the data show that the chronicity of grief itself does not seem to mediate the occurrence of complicated grief reactions. However, a close aggregation of losses, as well as discrimination, homophobia, low social support, lack of partner recognition for financial benefits and medical care rights, and greater difficulties in resocialization than those experienced in the general population are well known to increase the deleterious impact of bereavement among MSMs. Although most depressive symptoms experienced after bereavement are transient,[41] a significant sub-group eventually develops bereavement-associated MDD.

Grief is now typically designated as involving 2 types of affective processes: depressed mood and traumatic distress (with avoidance and intrusions). Yet, separation distress as a third type of affective process might be the most prominent type of distress in bereavement vis-à-vis the occurrence of complicated grief reactions. Separation distress refers to a set of symptoms with direct relationship to the loss as the organizing factor (eg, having difficulty acknowledging the death; assuming symptoms related to the deceased person; and experiencing excessive irritability, bitterness, or anger related to the death). Of note regarding bereavement, an RCT conducted with HIV-positive and HIV-negative homosexual men experiencing a loss over the prior 6 months who were randomly assigned to a semi-structured group intervention (with groups separated by HIV status) showed a significant effect on overall psychological distress and specifically on grief level when compared with community standard-of-care, bereaved control participants.[42] Moreover, the effects persisted when control variables were applied. In addition, an ad hoc complicated grief index that was analyzed in that study showed a significant intervention condition reduction for both HIV-positive and HIV-negative individuals. Ultimately, it seems that supportive therapy for grief may not be necessary (but may nevertheless prove helpful) in cases of uncomplicated grief. However, supportive interventions, particularly those developed specifically for complicated grief reactions,[43] may be critical to provide for future functioning. Resilience may not only be attained but also may be promoted through intervention.[44] The purview of end-of-life care for those with HIV/AIDS should also be extended beyond the sphere of the patient to the deceased patient's loved ones and social support network. Thus, such interventions might not only be targeted to ameliorate the negative impact of bereavement (eg, reduction of the allostatic stress load of chronic loss burden) but also to extend beyond such targets to treat to a target of positive mental health and true wellness. The use of established stress management interventions together with social support groups and coping skills enhancement training could be used to achieve such a goal in the future.

SYNTHESIS AND SUMMARY

The HIV/AIDS epidemic has changed perhaps more dramatically than any other disease over as short a period of time since its initial description. The Centers for Disease Control and Prevention (CDC) began tracking cases of AIDS in 1981, and there was no direct treatment of HIV infection whatsoever until 1987, when the US Food and Drug Administration approved zidovudine (then called azidothymidine). Since that time, the number of ARVs has mushroomed, and the ability to monitor and control the progression of the disease has made amazing strides. Morbidity and mortality from HIV/AIDS has been tremendously reduced in high-resource countries. This article reviews the current status of end-of-life care issues in HIV/AIDS. Although the progress in the treatment of the disease has been impressive and the projected life span for infected patients has been greatly increased, the impact of these developments is felt differently around the world.

This article reports on the end-of-life care issues in HIV/AIDS as a stage-like, yet overlapping process in which the patients generally start with the diagnosis, in which the focus is primary medical care to suppress plasma viral load to non-detectable levels and deter the development of any symptoms. Eventually, a subgroup of symptoms do occur and predominate that do not reflect any specific HIV-associated disease but rather the generalized progression of HIV infection itself. This is the stage of palliative care characterized by the symptoms of fatigue, pain, insomnia, decreased libido and hypogonadism, decreased memory, and concentration (HAND), depression, and distorted body image. Next, the stage of hospice care is discussed from a historical vantage point related to its current status. Then how the stage of hospice care leads directly to entry into the death and dying process and the prominent issues that are frequently neglected in that end-of-life stage were discussed. Finally, the typical endpoint for the discussion of end-of-life care issues is taken a step beyond the usual framework to consider the impact of the death of the patient on others; that is, the potent impact of bereavement on a patient's loved ones and entire social support network. With this depiction, it is hoped that preparation for and treatment of end-of-life care issues will not only be undertaken as clinically adeptly as was done in times past but will also be better informed by the development of the end-of-life literature to the present day.

ACKNOWLEDGMENTS

This work was contributed to by the following National Institute of Mental Health grants to Dr K. Goodkin: MH48628, MH48628S, and MH53802.

REFERENCES

1. Murphy EL, Collier AC, Kalish LA, et al. Highly active antiretroviral therapy decreases mortality and morbidity in patients with advanced HIV disease. Ann Intern Med 2001;135:17–26.
2. Barroso J, Harmon JL, Madison JL, et al. Intensity, chronicity, circumstances, and consequences of HIV-related fatigue: a longitudinal study. Clin Nurs Res 2014; 23(5):514–28.
3. Barichello T, Simões LR, Generoso JS, et al. Erythropoietin prevents cognitive impairment and oxidative parameters in Wistar rats subjected to pneumococcal meningitis. Transl Res 2014;163(5):503–13.
4. Rabkin JG, McElhiney MC, Rabkin R. Treatment of HIV-related fatigue with armodafinil: a placebo-controlled randomized trial. Psychosomatics 2011;52(4): 328–36.
5. Hewitt DJ, McDonald M, Portenoy RK, et al. Pain syndromes and etiologies in ambulatory AIDS patients. Pain 1997;70:117–23.
6. Parker R, Stein DJ, Jelsma J. Pain in people living with HIV/AIDS: a systematic review. J Int AIDS Soc 2014;17:18719.
7. Edelman EJ, Gordon K, Becker WC, et al. Receipt of opioid analgesics by HIV-infected and uninfected patients. J Gen Intern Med 2013;28(1):82–90.
8. Rubinstein ML, Selwyn PA. High prevalence of insomnia in an outpatient population with HIV infection. J Acquir Immune Defic Syndr Hum Retrovirol 1998;19: 260–5.
9. Clifford DB, Evans S, Yang Y, et al. Impact of efavirenz on neuropsychological performance and symptoms in HIV-infected individuals. Ann Intern Med 2005; 143(10):714–21.
10. Eiden C, Peyriere H, Peytavin G, et al. Severe insomnia related to high concentrations of raltegravir. AIDS 2011;25(5):725–7.
11. Crum-Cianflone NF, Poehlman Roediger M, Moore DJ, et al. Prevalence and factors associated with sleep disturbances among early-treated HIV-infected persons. Clin Infect Dis 2012;54(10):1485–94.

12. Phillips KD, Skelton WD. Effects of individualized acupuncture on sleep quality in HIV disease. J Assoc Nurses AIDS Care 2001;12(1):27–39.

13. Toma S, Omonuwa BS, Goforth HW, et al. The pharmacologic management of insomnia in patients with HIV. J Clin Sleep Med 2009;5(3):251–62.

14. Schlich C, Romanelli F. Issues surrounding testosterone replacement therapy. Hosp Pharm 2016;51(9):712–20.

15. Antinori A, Arendt G, Becker JT, et al. Updated research nosology for HIV- associated neurocognitive disorders (HAND). Neurology 2007;69:1789–99.

16. Milanini B, Wendelken LA, Esmaeili-Firidouni P, et al. The Montreal cognitive assessment to screen for cognitive impairment in HIV patients older than 60 years. J Acquir Immune Defic Syndr 2014;67(1):67–70.

17. Power C, Selnes OA, Grim JA, et al. HIV dementia scale: a rapid screening test. J Acquir Immune Defic Syndr 1995;8:273–8.

18. Sacktor NC, Wong M, Nakasujja N, et al. The International HIV Dementia Scale: a new rapid screening test for HIV dementia. AIDS 2005;19(13):1367–74.

19. Goodkin K, Hardy DJ, Singh D, et al. Diagnostic utility of the International HIV Dementia Scale for HIV-associated neurocognitive impairment and disorder in South Africa. J Neuropsychiatry Clin Neurosci 2014;26:352–8.

20. Marin-Webb V, Jessen H, Kopp U, et al. Validation of the International HIV dementia scale as a screening tool for HIV-associated neurocognitive disorders in a German-speaking HIV outpatient clinic. PLoS One 2016;11(12):e0168225.

21. Wu AW, Rubin HR, Mathews WC, et al. A health status questionnaire using 30 items from the Medical Outcomes Study. Med Care 1991;29:786–98.

22. Abrass CK, Appelbaum J, Boyd CM, et al. Updated. The HIV and Aging Consensus Project. Recommended treatment strategies for clinicians managing older patients with HIV. Washington, DC: American Academy of HIV Medicine; 2014. p. 88.

23. Simoni JM, Safren SA, Manhart LE, et al. Challenges in addressing depression in HIV research: assessment, cultural context, and methods. AIDS Behav 2011; 15(2):376–88.

24. Sacktor N, Skolasky RL, Haughey N, et al. Paroxetine and fluconazole therapy for HAND: a double-blind, placebo-controlled trial. Conference on Retroviruses and Opportunistic Infections (CROI). Boston, February 22–25, 2016. Abstract 146.

25. Evans DL, Ten Have TR, Douglas SD, et al. Association of depression with viral load, CD8 T lymphocytes, and natural killer cells in women with HIV infection. Am J Psychiatry 2002;159(10):1752–9.

26. Martinez P, Tsai AC, Muzoora C, et al. Reversal of the kynurenine pathway of tryptophan catabolism may improve depression in ART-treated HIV-infected Ugandans. J Acquir Immune Defic Syndr 2014;65(4):456–62.

27. Collins E, Wagner C, Walmsley S. Psychosocial impact of the lipodystrophy syndrome in HIV infection. AIDS Read 2000;10(9):546–50.

28. Alencastro PR, Barcellos NT, Wolff FH, et al. People living with HIV on ART have accurate perception of lipodystrophy signs: a cross-sectional study. BMC Res Notes 2017;10(1):40.

29. Blashill AJ, Safren SA, Wilhelm S, et al. Cognitive behavioral therapy for body image and self-care (CBT-BISC) in sexual minority men living with HIV: a randomized controlled trial. Health Psychol 2017. https://doi.org/10.1037/hea0000505.

30. Brown TT, Glesby MJ. Management of the metabolic effects of HIV and HIV drugs. Nat Rev Endocrinol 2011;8(1):11–21.

31. Sheth SH, Larson RJ. The efficacy and safety of insulin-sensitizing drugs in HIV-associated lipodystrophy syndrome: a meta-analysis of randomized trials. BMC Infect Dis 2010;10:183.

32. Nelson L, Stewart KJ. Plastic surgical options for HIV-associated lipodystrophy. J Plast Reconstr Aesthet Surg 2008;61(4):359–65.

33. Slomka J, Prince-Paul M, Webel A, et al. palliative care, hospice, and advance care planning: views of people living with HIV and other chronic conditions. J Assoc Nurses AIDS Care 2016;27(4):476–84.

34. Shorthill J, DeMarco RF. The relevance of palliative care in HIV and aging. Interdiscip Top Gerontol Geriatr 2017;42:222–33.

35. Hold JL, Blake BJ, Byrne M, et al. Opening life's gifts: facing death for a second time. J Assoc Nurses AIDS Care 2017. https://doi.org/10.1016/j.jana.2017.03.011.

36. Delpech V, Lundgren J. Death from AIDS is preventable, so why are people still dying of AIDS in Europe? Euro Surveill 2014;19(47):20973.

37. Mallinson RK. Grief in the context of HIV: recommendations for practice. J Assoc Nurses AIDS Care 2013;24(1 Suppl):S61–71.

38. Goforth HW, Lowery J, Cutson TM, et al. Impact of bereavement on progression of AIDS and HIV infection: a review. Psychosomatics 2009;50(5):433–9.

39. Summers J, Zisook S, Atkinson JH, et al. Psychiatric morbidity with acquired immune deficiency-related grief resolution. J Nerv Ment Dis 1995;183:384–9.

40. Zisook S, Shuchter SR. Depression through the first year after the death of a spouse. Am J Psychiatry 1991;148:1346–52.

41. Wortman CB, Silver RC. The myths of coping with loss. J Consult Clin Psychol 1989;57:349–57.

42. Goodkin K, Blaney NT, Feaster DJ, et al. A randomized controlled trial of a bereavement support group intervention in human immunodeficiency virus type 1-seropositive and seronegative homosexual men. Arch Gen Psychiatry 1999; 55(1):52–9.

43. Shear K, Frank E, Houck PR, et al. Treatment of complicated grief: a randomized controlled trial. JAMA 2005;293(21):2601–8.

44. Yu NX, Chan CL, Zhang J, et al. Resilience and vulnerability: prolonged grief in the bereaved spouses of marital partners who died of AIDS. AIDS Care 2016; 28(4):441–4.

Moving?

Make sure your subscription moves with you!

To notify us of your new address, find your **Clinics Account Number** (located on your mailing label above your name), and contact customer service at:

Email: journalscustomerservice-usa@elsevier.com

800-654-2452 (subscribers in the U.S. & Canada)
314-447-8871 (subscribers outside of the U.S. & Canada)

Fax number: 314-447-8029

Elsevier Health Sciences Division
Subscription Customer Service
3251 Riverport Lane
Maryland Heights, MO 63043

Moving?

Make sure your subscription moves with you!

To notify us of your new address, find your Clinics Account number (located on your mailing label above your name), and contact customer service at:

Email: journalscustomerservice-usa@elsevier.com

800-654-2452 (subscribers in the U.S. & Canada)
314-447-8871 (subscribers outside of the U.S. & Canada)

Fax number: 314-447-8029

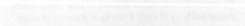

Elsevier Health Sciences Division
Subscription Customer Service
3251 Riverport Lane
Maryland Heights, MO 63043

*Please notify us at least 4 weeks in advance of move.

Printed and bound by CPI Group (UK) Ltd, Croydon, CR0 4YY

03/10/2024

01040388-0010